THE NEW
PEOPLE
·NOT PATIENTS·

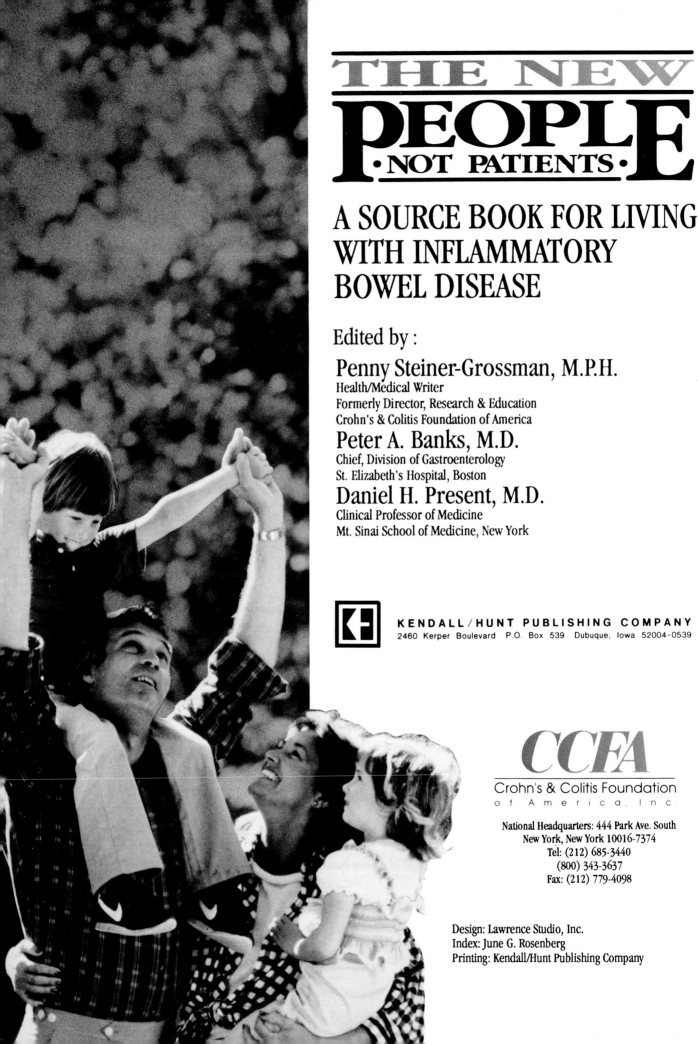

THE NEW
PEOPLE
·NOT PATIENTS·

A SOURCE BOOK FOR LIVING WITH INFLAMMATORY BOWEL DISEASE

Edited by :

Penny Steiner-Grossman, M.P.H.
Health/Medical Writer
Formerly Director, Research & Education
Crohn's & Colitis Foundation of America

Peter A. Banks, M.D.
Chief, Division of Gastroenterology
St. Elizabeth's Hospital, Boston

Daniel H. Present, M.D.
Clinical Professor of Medicine
Mt. Sinai School of Medicine, New York

KENDALL/HUNT PUBLISHING COMPANY
2460 Kerper Boulevard P.O. Box 539 Dubuque, Iowa 52004-0539

CCFA
Crohn's & Colitis Foundation
of America, Inc.

National Headquarters: 444 Park Ave. South
New York, New York 10016-7374
Tel: (212) 685-3440
(800) 343-3637
Fax: (212) 779-4098

Design: Lawrence Studio, Inc.
Index: June G. Rosenberg
Printing: Kendall/Hunt Publishing Company

Contributors

Peter A. Banks, M.D.
St. Elizabeth's Hospital
Boston, Massachusetts

Theodore M. Bayless, M.D.
Johns Hopkins Medical Institutions
Baltimore, Maryland

Philip S. Bentlif, M.D.
Kelsey-Seybold Clinic
Houston, Texas

Jason Bodzin, M.D.
Sinai Hospital
Detroit, Michigan

Gregory F. Bonner, M.D.
Cleveland Clinic Florida
Ft. Lauderdale, Florida

Lawrence J. Brandt, M.D.
Montefiore Medical Center
Bronx, New York

Robert Burakoff, M.D.
Winthrop University Hospital
Mineola, New York

Fredric Daum, M.D.
North Shore University Hospital
Manhasset, New York

Douglas A. Drossman, M.D.
University of North Carolina
Chapel Hill, North Carolina

Mary-Joan Gerson, Ph.D.
Mt. Sinai Medical Center
New York, New York

Stephen B. Hanauer, M.D.
The University of Chicago
Chicago, Illinois

Jeffrey S. Hyams, M.D.
Hartford Hospital
Hartford, Connecticut

Henry D. Janowitz, M.D.
Mt. Sinai Medical Center
New York, New York

Marvin Kaplan, M.D.
Lenox Hill Hospital
New York, New York

Barbara S. Kirschner, M.D.
The University of Chicago
Chicago, Illinois

Burton I. Korelitz, M.D.
Lenox Hill Hospital
New York, New York

Audrey Kron, M.A.
Center for Coping with Chronic Illness
Detroit, Michigan

Marvin Lieberman, Ph.D.
New York Academy of Medicine
New York, New York

Robin S. McLeod, M.D.
Mt. Sinai Hospital
Toronto, Ontario, Canada

Joel F. Panish, M.D.
Los Angeles Gastroenterology
Medical Group
Los Angeles, California

Mark A. Peppercorn, M.D.
Beth Israel Hospital
Boston, Massachusetts

Daniel H. Present, M.D.
Mt. Sinai Medical Center
New York, New York

Jane W. Present, M.A.
Crohn's & Colitis Foundation of
America
New York, New York

Jerome I. Rotter, M.D.
Cedars-Sinai Medical Center
Los Angeles, California

William Ruderman, M.D.
Cleveland Clinic Florida
Ft. Lauderdale, Florida

David B. Sachar, M.D.
Mt. Sinai Medical Center
New York, New York

Penny Steiner-Grossman, M.P.H.
Health/Medical Writer
Brooklyn, New York

Julianne Stroud, R.N., C.E.T.
Mt. Carmel/Mercy Hospital
Detroit, Michigan

Marjorie M. Sutton, M.S., R.D.
The University of Chicago
Chicago, Illinois

Stephan R. Targan, M.D.
University of California
Los Angeles, California

Contents

Preface

In planning the first edition of this book during the mid-1980's, we tried to give people with IBD the tools to become self-advocates. To accomplish this they would need a source book with sufficient information to help them understand their diseases, learn about their legal rights, and begin to fight back. We enlisted the help of many individuals who shared our philosophy and purpose.

We have now lived through the decade of the 80's, with its messages of self-fulfillment, fitness, and wellness. It is heartening to see so many Americans adopting healthier life styles—engaging in vigorous exercise, eating healthy foods, quitting smoking. Nevertheless, the wellness message sometimes makes us feel that we, and we alone, are responsible for maintaining our health and avoiding illness. Unfortunately for people with IBD, and people with any chronic illness, healthy behavior doesn't always lead to good health. So how do we adapt the "wellness" message to suit the realities of having inflammatory bowel disease?

Unfortunately for people with IBD, and people with any chronic illness, healthy behavior doesn't always lead to good health.

Wellness for the person with IBD means coping in the face of pain, discomfort, and lack of energy. It means maintaining a positive outlook while still worrying about being a burden to others, struggling to find health insurance coverage, and just getting through each day. But while control over health is not always possible, with improved IBD treatments there is abundant room for most of the good things life has to offer: family, friendship, intimacy, physical activity, the enjoyment of good food and good times. Our "wellness" message for the 1990's is that, despite limited control over our health, we are still people, not patients.

We had the help of many people in preparing this book: physicians, psychologists, nurses, other health professionals, and the people whose stories allow us glimpses of the reality of living with IBD. In addition, we want to thank Shirley Howard for her patience in preparing the manuscript; writers Barbara Rosenstein, Paul Tarricone, and Michael Kennedy, who provided some of the material in Chapters 9 and 10 as well as some of the biographical sketches; Roy Temkin of Chase/Temkin & Associates for providing the line drawings; June Rosenberg for preparing the index; and James V. Romano, CCFA's Director of Research and Education, for his encouragement and support of this project.

In addition, we thank Sandoz Pharmaceuticals for making possible the printing of this book. Through their generosity, we will be able to reach many thousands of people with IBD who need the information contained in these pages.

Lastly, we thank you, our readers, the people with IBD, your families and loved ones. We hope you will learn as much from this book as we continue to learn from you.

Penny Steiner-Grossman
Peter A. Banks
Daniel H. Present

Foreword

I am delighted to inform people with inflammatory bowel disease of the beginning of a new era in our search to understand these conditions. Building on significant scientific advances made during the last part of the 1980's, the Crohn's & Colitis Foundation of America (CCFA) has declared the 1990's "The Decade of the Cure." To ensure our success, we have embarked on a program called "Challenges in IBD Research: Agenda for the 1990's." This international program is by far the most coordinated effort to date and is designed to apply all that is currently known to the questions about IBD that remain unanswered.

As people with IBD, you have a most important role in this new agenda. If we learned anything from the 1980's, the so-called "me decade," it was to pay attention to our bodies and our health, and to trust ourselves to take care of ourselves. This also applies to people with illnesses like IBD, but it doesn't mean that you are alone with this responsibility. It means that you have the right to know everything about your condition and to expect that physicians and other caregivers should do everything in their power to aid you in this task. It wasn't long ago that people with IBD were fearful of asking questions and were expected to be satisified with what little information they were given. No more. The information generated from a healthy dialogue between you and your physician can actually improve your care and augment the data resources for future IBD research.

It wasn't long ago that people with IBD were fearful of asking questions and were expected to be satisified with what little information they were given.

While we are looking for the cure, we are striving to improve treatments. What we now know about the nature of these diseases has allowed us to target new drugs to interfere with the inflammatory process.

Some older medications have been revised and updated so that they have fewer side-effects and are easier to tolerate. New medications are on the horizon and will be brought to you as quickly as possible. We now know that subtle differences exist within general disease categories. For example, there is new genetic evidence suggesting the existence of at least two subtypes of ulcerative colitis. More information on the unique characteristics of IBD will continue to result in more useful ways of treating these diseases.

Among the things you can do to help yourself and other people with IBD is to get involved. Talk about your feelings and your experiences with other people with IBD. Begin to educate yourself, your family, and the people who share your life. Learn about treatments, but also learn about the many ways you can help yourself to feel better. You can also teach people about what you face, how your life is affected. Teach your doctor about your symptoms, your feelings, and about your special needs.

Support groups for people with IBD began just over 10 years ago with a handful of groups in a few cities. Now there are hundreds of groups across the country. You can learn from people who cope well with their disease, and you can teach others how to cope as well as you do. There is nothing you can't do. That means everything from getting the job you want to feeling successful about your life. There are artists, bankers, doctors, athletes, and actors with IBD. There are also mothers, fathers, brothers, sisters, husbands, wives, boyfriends and girlfriends. Other people with IBD will encourage you to identify your goals and will help you see new ways to achieve them. Don't be afraid to share. The more people there are who know about IBD, the more people there are to care that a cure is eventually found.

We hope that you will use this new edition of **People . . . not Patients** as a guide for you, your family, your friends, your boss, teacher, and anyone you would like to know more about you. And remember, any questions which this book brings to mind are worth asking and deserve an answer. In the meantime, we will continue our efforts to solve the problem.

Stephan R. Targan, M.D.
Chairman, National Scientific Advisory Committee

Part I

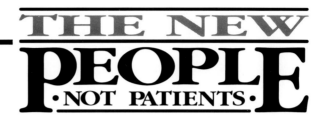

Understanding Your Illness

About Inflammatory Bowel Disease

The diseases we call Crohn's disease and ulcerative colitis have been given the convenient label "inflammatory bowel disease" (IBD) as if to emphasize their differences. There *are* important differences: Crohn's disease may affect any part of the bowel from mouth to anus while ulcerative colitis attacks only the colon; Crohn's disease involves the full thickness of bowel wall while ulcerative colitis inflames only the inner lining; ulcerative colitis is cured by surgery while Crohn's disease is not. Crohn's disease has increased dramatically in incidence over the past few decades while ulcerative colitis has remained relatively stable. These are important differences, but at the present time, the similarities between the two diseases appear to overshadow the differences. This may be changing, however, as scientists begin to look for different types of Crohn's disease and different types of ulcerative colitis.

At the present time, the similarities between the two diseases appear to overshadow the differences. This may be changing, however, as scientists begin to look for different types of Crohn's disease and different types of ulcerative colitis.

Both types of IBD occur predominantly in Western or developed countries of the world, especially Scandinavia, England, Western Europe, Israel and the United States. In recent years, IBD is being reported in Japan. Conversely, IBD is rarely detected in peoples of Africa, most of Asia and parts of South America, areas of poor sanitation and lower nutritional standards. Although all ages are at risk for IBD, the greatest risk seems to be between the ages 10 and 20, with relatively equal division between the sexes. Crohn's disease and ulcerative colitis tend to cluster in some families, although a specific genetic pattern has not yet been identified. Up to 20 percent of people with IBD may have one or more relatives with either disease.

The purpose of this introductory chapter is to summarize current knowledge about both forms of IBD, with special emphasis on the nature of the inflammatory process they have in common, and on the search for a cause.

The Organs of the Gastrointestinal Tract

In order to understand the nature of IBD, it is first necessary to review the organs of the gastrointestinal (GI) tract and to understand the way they function. The best way to picture the GI tract, or gut, is as a continuous tube which begins at the mouth and ends at the anus (See diagram). This tube is actually *outside* the body proper, because both ends are open to the external environment. Its chief functions, as we know, are to allow nutrients to enter and wastes to pass out of the body, and to

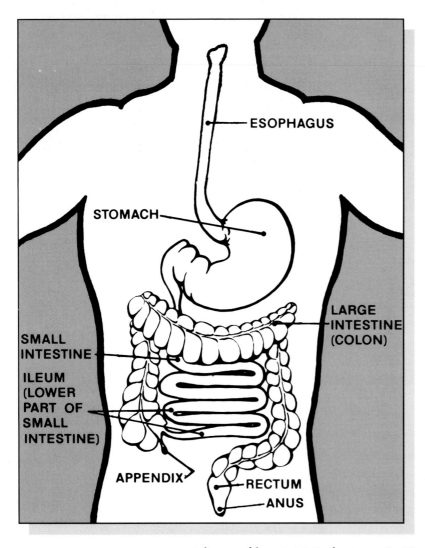

ESOPHAGUS

STOMACH

LARGE
INTESTINE
(COLON)

SMALL
INTESTINE

ILEUM
(LOWER
PART OF
SMALL
INTESTINE)

APPENDIX

RECTUM

ANUS

A diagram of the gastrointestinal system, or "gut."

protect the body from infection through a complex network of immune cells.

The parts of the digestive tube as shown in the diagram in descending order are the mouth, esophagus, stomach, small intestine (duodenum, jejunum and ileum), large intestine (colon), rectum and anus. The continuous tube that forms these varied organs is arranged in layers, and these layers make up the **bowel wall.** The innermost layer of the bowel wall is called the **mucosa,** or mucous membrane layer. Inside the bowel wall is the hollow space or **lumen,** which contains the food we eat in its various stages of digestion. As food passes through the lumen, the various **accessory organs**—the salivary glands, liver, gallbladder and pancreas— empty their secretions to aid in digestion.

The "Gut" as an Immune Organ

The second—and much less understood function of the GI tract—is to protect the body against invasion by harmful or toxic substances. The mucosal layer of intestine which serves to absorb nutrients also contains many types of immune cells which act as defenders in recognizing foreign substances **(antigens)** and preventing them from crossing the mucosal barrier and entering the body. Some of these cells **(macrophages** and **mast cells)** act by engulfing the harmful materials; others, such as **lymphocytes,** produce antibodies which bind to and neutralize these antigens, bacteria or viruses. This usually efficient system—allowing the billions of bacteria and viruses to exist in the intestinal lumen without damaging the body—is a perfect illustration of the intestine as an organ "outside" the body.

The Inflammatory Response in IBD

Sometimes the mucosal immune barrier breaks down, resulting in entry of harmful bacteria or other materials into deeper layers of intestine. This sets up an inflammatory reaction which results in **edema** (swelling), increased blood flow, and **ulcerations** (disruptions in the intestinal lining) such as those seen in ulcerative colitis. These ulcerations may penetrate deep into the bowel wall and involve the full thickness of intestine. This is the type of lesion caused by Crohn's disease.

When healing occurs, the gut may become fibrous or scarred around the areas that were previously inflamed. This may cause a narrowing of the bowel, or **stricture,** which could lead to partial or total obstruction of intestinal flow.

The Search for a Possible Cause

Some scientists feel that the immune response observed in IBD is a chronic state of inflammation, initiated by an unknown antigen and perpetuated by constant leakage of bacterial products through the wounded bowel wall. Others suggest that the inflammatory cells are reacting to the IBD patient's own tissues as if they were foreign, a process we know as **autoimmunity.** At the very least, we do know that certain specific disturbances have been found in persons with IBD. These findings do not prove an immune origin for IBD, but they do raise important questions that need to be answered. Are the immune disturbances seen in IBD patients the cause of the ailment, or are they an exaggerated response

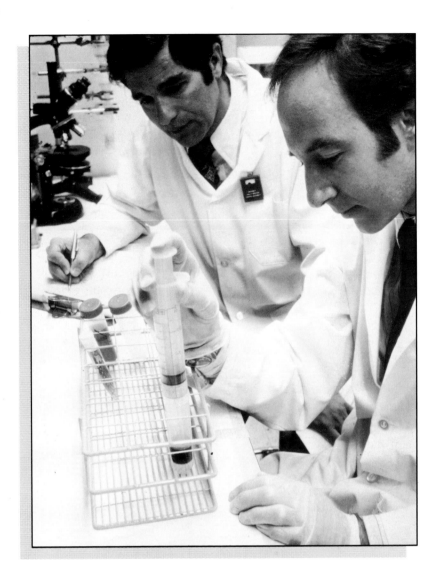

to an agent we have not yet located? If IBD is found to be caused by an infectious agent, isn't there still a disturbance in the immune response that prevents some people from overcoming the infection and subjects them to a chronic disease that lasts a lifetime?

Much has been learned about the patterns of inflammatory bowel disease in the past 60 years, not all of which could be contained within this chapter. Even though the cause has not yet been identified, people with IBD are capable of leading long, useful and often comfortable lives with careful medical and surgical management. Hopefully, expanding research programs such as those sponsored by the Crohn's & Colitis Foundation of America will lead to the identification of the causative agents and to the eventual eradication of this group of diseases. In the meantime, we must learn as much as possible about IBD, the demands it makes on our living patterns, and the ways we can learn to cope with those demands. These are the reasons for this book.

Diagnostic Procedures and Laboratory Tests in IBD

2

During an evaluation for inflammatory bowel disease, features of both the initial history and physical examination can suggest problems that often require confirmation with the use of specific diagnostic tests. Diagnostic procedures and laboratory tests necessary for the evaluation of inflammatory bowel disease can be categorized in the following way: (1) blood and urine tests; (2) stool examinations; (3) radiological procedures; and (4) endoscopic procedures

This chapter will provide some basic explanations about why specific tests may be ordered, and how these tests are useful for the diagnosis and management of IBD. An explanation of how these radiologic and endoscopic procedures are performed will help you prepare for and understand the diagnostic studies ordered by your physician.

Blood and Urine Tests

There are no blood or urine tests that are *specific* for the diagnosis of IBD. However, there are several blood tests that can be useful in suggesting the presence of IBD, and in assessing disease activity. For the most part, there is no preparation for these tests. However, your doctor may ask you to fast for such tests as a blood sugar evaluation, or cholesterol and triglyceride determinations.

A **complete blood count** includes a measurement of the hemoglobin, hematocrit, white blood cell count, and differential. The hemoglobin (Hb or Hgb) and hematocrit (Hct) levels are used to determine the presence of anemia. In IBD there can be multiple causes of anemia, such as bleeding, vitamin or mineral deficiencies, or the ongoing destruction of red blood cells (RBCs). The white blood count (WBC) is elevated by active IBD or by the presence of infectious complications of IBD, such as an abdominal abscess. The use of steroid preparations like prednisone can also increase the white blood cell count without indicating active disease. The differential count can be obtained to measure the proportion of the different types of white blood cells present within the blood. Inflammation and infection cause an increase in the number of immature white blood cells released by the bone marrow into the blood. This increase in immature white blood cells can be detected on the differential count.

The **erythrocyte sedimentation rate (ESR)** is a useful test for measuring the presence of active inflammation or infection. It tends to be elevated during a flare-up in the activity of inflammatory bowel disease.

The presence of anemia, an elevated white blood cell count, and increased erythrocyte sedimentation rate are all *indirect* evidence suggesting the presence of active disease. In a person with known inflammatory bowel disease, these tests can be used to monitor disease activity and response to treatment.

Tests Commonly Performed in IBD

Blood and Urine Tests

1. Complete blood count (CBC)
2. Erythrocyte sedimentation rate (ESR)
3. Prothrombin time
4. Blood chemistries
5. Schilling test
6. Urinalysis and/or urine culture

Stool Examinations

1. Occult blood
2. White blood cells (WBCs)
3. Culture and sensitivity (C&S)
4. Ova and parasites
5. *Clostridium difficile* toxin

Radiologic Procedures

1. Barium enema examination (BE)
2. Upper GI and small bowel follow-through
3. Enteroclysis
4. Diagnostic ultrasound
5. Abdominal CT scan
6. Magnetic resonance imaging (MRI)

Endoscopic Procedures

1. Sigmoidoscopy (with biopsy)
2. Colonoscopy (with biopsy)
3. Upper gastrointestinal endoscopy (with biopsy)

Coagulation tests are performed to provide information about clotting ability. The prothrombin time may be prolonged in people with IBD as a result of impaired intestinal absorption of vitamin K, poor nutrition, or prolonged use of antibiotics. The **platelet count,** a test measuring the number of cells involved in blood clotting, is also raised when there is active inflammation or infection.

Multiple tests called **blood chemistries,** available on complex analyzers, provide information about nutritional status and general health, body electrolyte balance, and liver and kidney function. Serum cholesterol, total protein, and albumin are all indirect measures of nutritional status. Blood electrolytes include sodium, potassium, chloride, and bicarbonate, calcium, phosphorous, and magnesium and can be abnormal as a result of impaired absorption, diarrhea, or dehydration. Liver function tests include a bilirubin level, alkaline phosphatase, and specific liver enzyme tests (AST and ALT). Finally, blood urea nitrogen (BUN) and creatinine levels are simple and accurate tests to measure kidney function. These tests are widely available and are performed using blood obtained from a simple venipuncture. Often they are performed as part of a chemistry examination known as a **sequential multiple analysis (SMA)** profile. Severe diarrhea can cause abnormalities of the blood electrolytes or dehydration; these will be reflected in abnormalities of kidney function. Blood chemistries reflecting nutritional status also tend to be lower in individuals with active IBD.

Anemia caused by IBD may result from diminished levels of vitamin B-12, folate, or iron. These can be caused by improper absorption in active Crohn's disease. Loss of blood from the intestinal tract in active IBD can result in iron deficiency anemia. Vitamin B-12 deficiency can occur in patients with active Crohn's disease involving the terminal ileum or in those who have had surgical resection of their terminal ileum. A **Schilling test** can be performed to measure abnormalities of the absorption of vitamin B-12. A radiolabeled vitamin B-12 preparation is taken by mouth and the blood and urine B-12 levels are measured over the next several hours. Low folate levels can be found when there is malnutrition caused by active Crohn's disease, or as a result of taking sulfasalazine.

A **urinalysis** is performed to look for bacteria or blood cells in the urine. Bacterial infections of the urine can occur in IBD as a result of kidney stones, or formation of fistulas between the intestine and bladder.

Stool Examinations

Intestinal infections may mimic inflammatory bowel disease and can cause fever, diarrhea, abdominal cramping, and sometimes nausea and vomiting. Since some intestinal infections can mimic ulcerative colitis or Crohn's disease, stool studies are important in differentiating inflammatory bowel disease from other conditions. Even in those people with known IBD, the development of diarrhea, fever, or abdominal discomfort can result from a superimposed infection rather than from a worsening of the IBD.

Stool samples can be collected by the patient in a special container or will sometimes be obtained by the physician at the time of a rectal examination or sigmoidoscopy. Laxatives or enemas should not be taken prior to the collection of stool samples to avoid irritating the lining of the bowel, destroying certain parasites, and diluting white blood cells in the specimen. Stool specimens are examined for the presence of microscopic amounts of hidden blood **(occult blood)** using a special test card which your doctor can supply together

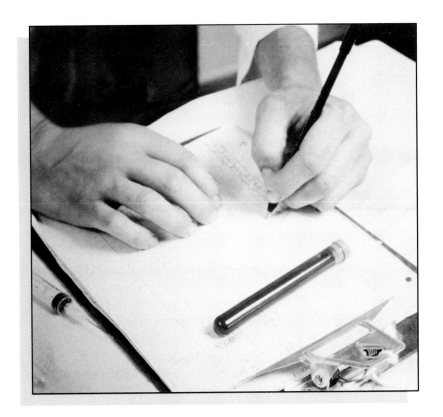

with a developing agent. After staining, a stool specimen can also be examined for white blood cells under the microscope. Blood and white blood cells are found in the stool either in active IBD or in bacterial infections of the bowel, as well as in other conditions.

Bacterial infections can also mimic both ulcerative colitis and Crohn's disease.

Amebiasis and **giardiasis** are parasitic conditions that can mimic the symptoms of IBD. Using concentrating techniques, stool can be tested for the presence of various intestinal parasites **(ova and parasites).** Since parasite shedding in the stool can be an intermittent process, you may need to provide several stool specimens at different times to eliminate the possibility of a parasitic infection. Blood tests can also be performed to verify a diagnosis of amebiasis.

Bacterial infections can also mimic both ulcerative colitis and Crohn's disease. Your doctor may send stool specimens for culture of such bacterial organisms as *Salmonella, Shigella, Campylobacter,* or *Yersinia.* This test is called a **culture and sensitivity (C&S).** The use of broad-spectrum antibiotics can sometimes allow the overgrowth of an organism known as *Clostridium difficile.* This organism can cause a form of colitis at times indistinguishable from ulcerative colitis. Stool specimens can be tested for the presence of a toxin secreted by this bacterial organism, and specific treatment can be given to eradicate this problem.

Radiologic Procedures

A **barium enema** examination is often used during the initial evaluation of IBD or to determine when complications such as strictures have developed. It is usually possible to visualize the junction of the small bowel and the colon known as the terminal ileum. Active inflammation in this region of the small bowel is common in Crohn's disease, and can be identified by this examination. To prepare for a barium enema, it is necessary to empty the colon of stool to allow barium to coat its inner surface. You may be asked to take a clear liquid diet, oral laxatives the day before the procedure, and rectal suppositories or enemas the morning of the procedure. An enema tube is inserted into the rectum. Barium is introduced through the enema tube, coating the mucosal lining of the colon. The radiologist can often differentiate between ulcerative colitis and Crohn's disease based on various features of the x-rays that are taken. However, a definitive diagnosis is often not possible, and colonoscopic examination, even up to and including the terminal ileum, may be needed. Both barium enema and colonoscopy can be dangerous in patients with severe or toxic colitis, and should not be performed under these circumstances.

Evaluation of the upper digestive tract can be performed by a radiologic procedure known as **upper gastrointestinal series** and **small bowel follow-through** examination. This test is performed when your physician needs to determine if there is inflammation or ulceration of the esophagus, stomach, or small intestine, and can be helpful in establishing an initial diagnosis of Crohn's disease. It can also be useful in detecting the presence of a stricture, (a narrowing of the bowel) or a fistula (a communicating tract of the bowel,) both of which can be complications of Crohn's disease. The test requires drinking a chalky liquid (usually available in strawberry or chocolate flavors) after which serial abdominal x-rays are obtained over two or more hours.

Another type of small bowel x-ray procedure is an **enteroclysis.** This is a specialized form of small bowel x-ray which provides fine detailed views of the lining of the small bowel. This test is specifically useful for detecting ulcerations or strictures of the small intestine. In this examination, a thin plastic tube is placed through the nose and directed under x-ray guidance into the small intestine. Barium mixed with air is then infused through this tube directly into the first portion of the small intestine. Your doctor may order this examination when small bowel disease is suspected, but cannot be defined by other techniques.

If obstruction of the small bowel is suspected, simple x-ray films of the abdomen are taken without the use of contrast agents. The presence of dilated loops of bowel with air and fluid within the intestine is helpful in defining the presence and extent of a bowel obstruction. Upper intestinal barium studies are usually *not* performed when obstruction is suspected; this is because barium is diluted by fluid retained in the narrowed bowel, making a precise diagnosis more difficult.

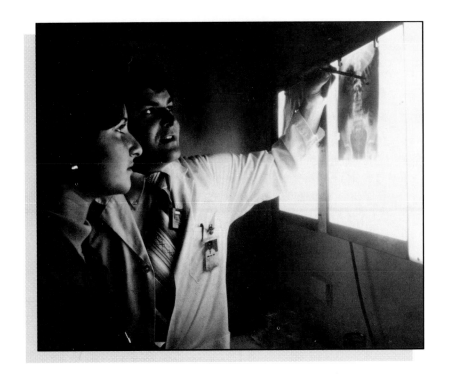

It is possible to examine many organs within the abdomen and pelvis using the technique of **diagnostic ultrasound.** Sound waves pass through the abdomen and encounter structures varying in wall thickness and fluid content, then bounce back to a recording device which visualizes the pattern of sound waves. This technique is considered "non-invasive" since it does not require the use of contrast material by mouth or vein and since there is no exposure to radiation. Ultrasound can detect the presence of gallstones and abscesses (collections of pus), both of which can complicate Crohn's disease. It is even possible for a radiologist to direct a thin tube, or a catheter, into an abdominal abscess under ultrasound guidance. The catheter can be used to drain the infected fluid collection, in the hope of eliminating the need for surgical drainage, at least temporarily. Ultrasound can also be used to determine whether an inflamed terminal

Exposure to X-Rays: How Much is Too Much?

Every time the physician orders an x-ray exam for a patient, he/she is making (or should be making) a risk vs. benefit decision: "Is the risk associated with this additional exposure of the patient to low level radiation *greater than* or *less than* the health benefits of the exam?" In the great majority of cases, the benefits to the patient far outweigh the risk of additional exposure. But among consumers and an increasing number of professionals, there is a growing concern that diagnostic x-rays may be misused, and that there are insufficient controls over the radiation exposure to patients during x-ray examinations.

What Happens During X-Ray Examination?

When a part of the human body is x-rayed, the rays are absorbed differently depending on the varying densities of body tissues. Denser tissues, such as bone, absorb the greatest number of x-rays and appear almost white on film. Softer tissues scatter the x-rays and appear gray, while air looks nearly black. In order to visualize clearly soft tissues like the intestine, bowel x-rays must use a **contrast medium** such as barium sulfate which absorbs and concentrates the x-rays, providing a clear image to facilitate diagnosis.

Obviously, the controlling factors in determining radiation exposure during x-ray exams are the number of exposures and the amount of radiation (rads) delivered with each exposure. According to standards set by the American College of Radiology, the goal in diagnostic x-rays must be to obtain the desired information using the smallest practical radiation exposure.

(continued on next page)

ileum is obstructing the right ureter and is causing swelling of the right kidney.

Computerized tomography (CT) scans can be used to evaluate organs within the body. This technique is performed in a special radiology unit with an x-ray machine capable of taking multiple, rapid views of portions of the body. Computerized data analysis is employed to reconstruct two dimensional "slices" of the body. This technique has revolutionized diagnostic imaging of the body and can provide exceptionally clear and detailed reproductions of internal organs. Although this techique can be complimentary to ultrasound evaluation, it is often used independently. Intravenous, oral, or rectally administered contrast material can be helpful in evaluating the liver, kidneys, and the intestine. Abdominal and pelvic CT scans are especially useful to allow insertion of needles or catheters into abscesses to facilitate drainage.

An **Indium scan** is a nuclear medicine study used to locate abscess or areas of active inflammation in IBD. This test is performed by attaching a radioactive tracer to white blood cells removed from the vein of a patient. These "labeled" cells are then re-injected back into the vein. A special machine that can detect radioactivity is used to scan the body for "hot spots" where the white blood cells accumulate in abnormal concentrations, usually in areas of infection or inflammation. The amount of radiation exposure experienced during an Indium scan is about the same as the radiation from two chest x-rays.

Sometimes Crohn's disease can be complicated by fistulas from the intestine to the skin around the rectum or to other places in the body. A **fistulagram** can be obtained by injecting the drainage site with a contrast medium; radiographs can then map the course of the fistula inside the body. When bowel inflammation causes obstruction or fistula formation to the urinary tract, your physician may order an **intravenous pyelogram (IVP)** examination. This requires the intravenous administration of iodine-containing contrast material which is excreted into the kidneys, ureters, and bladder. Outlines of the urinary tract can be obtained by radiographs taken at regular intervals.

Another radiologic procedure that is occasionally beneficial is a **magnetic resonance (MR) scan, or MRI.** This procedure uses a superconducting magnet to vibrate hydrogen molecules within the body. Signals emitted by these stimulated hydrogen molecules are then analyzed by computer to generate reconstructed images of the body in much the same way that CT scan images are created. An important difference between MR and CT imaging is that a CT scan requires the use of radiation, while MR testing only requires exposure to a high-powered but harmless magnetic field. Unfortunately, this technique has a limited role in evaluating the abdominal cavity. Your doctor may order this test to detect steroid-induced damage to the hips, or to evaluate fistulas, or abscesses, especially those located in the fatty or muscular tissues of the body.

Endoscopic Procedures

Endoscopy means looking at the inside of a hollow organ like the bowel through specially lighted tubes called **endoscopes.** These instruments can be passed through the rectum, the mouth, or even through small incisions in the abdominal wall to examine internal organs. **Sigmoidoscopy** (proctoscopy or proctosigmoidoscopy) is a commonly used procedure that can visualize the most distant portion of the colon including the rectum and sigmoid colon. Inspection of the lining of the intestine can be vitally important in diagnosing ulcerative colitis and in assessing disease activity or recurrence. Preparation usually involves the

(Continued from previous page)

Who is at Risk?

Some body parts are more sensitive to radiation than others. These include the breasts, thryoid gland, reproductive organs, and bone marrow. However, these areas are often not exposed during x-ray examination or they can be covered with special lead shields through which x-rays can't penetrate.

Obviously, individuals requiring frequent x-ray examinations are at the greatest risk of suffering ill effects from diagnostic x-rays. These include people with arthritic conditions, chronic heart or respiratory conditions, and gastrointesinal diseases like Crohn's disease and ulcerative colitis. In addition, some x-ray examinations such as upper GI series and barium enemas require the use of **fluoroscopy.** The radiologist will be present during the examination, following the course of the barium through your intestinal tract with a fluoroscope. This gives you a continuous x-ray exposure while it is functioning. This prolonged exposure may result from the inherent difficulty of performing the examination and the desire of the radiologist to provide your physician with the most complete information possible.

Since the effects of x-rays accumulate in the body over a lifetime, the greatest risk is to children with chronic conditions such as IBD. While these children *must* have timely x-ray examinations to monitor the course of illness over the years, no one knows how to calculate exactly what amount of low level radiation exposure poses a risk or threshold of danger.

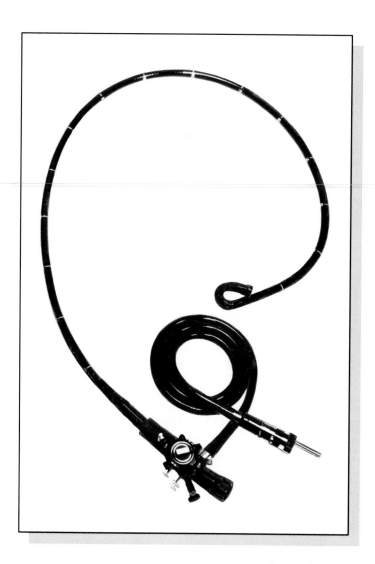

Fiberoptic colonoscope.

administration of one or more enemas. In an examination room designed for this procedure, your physician will first perform a rectal examination and then a flexible or rigid sigmoidoscope will be introduced into your rectum. The physician performing the procedure can see the lining of the lower colon, can assess the degree of inflammation, and can take biopsies (tissue samples), if necessary. Biopsies the size of a pencil point are obtained from the lining of the colon using a flexible forceps passed through a channel in the sigmoidoscope. These samples are then submitted to the pathology department in a fixative solution. These microscopic sections are then viewed by the pathologist. They provide information about the degree of inflammation and the presence of certain features suggesting a specific diagnosis, such as ulcerative colitis or Crohn's disease.

Colonoscopy allows the physician to examine the entire colon and often the terminal ileum. The gastroenterologist uses an instrument longer than the sigmoidoscope (see photo) which he/she introduces into the rectum and advances through the colon. This procedure takes longer than a sigmoidoscopy and generally requires the use of sedating medications such as Valium® (actually a muscle relaxant) and Demerol®. There are several reasons why a colonoscopy is performed in IBD. First, the physician needs to assess disease activity and extent of inflammation in individuals with disease of the colon. Second, since people with longstanding IBD are at an increased risk for developing colon cancer, surveillance colonoscopies can be performed at periodic intervals and random biopsies obtained to help exclude the presence of cancer or precancerous changes within the colon.

A number of problems can affect the upper digestive tract in patients with inflammatory bowel disease. Crohn's disease can affect any portion of the bowel including the upper intestine. Other problems may occur such as ulcer disease, reflux esophagitis, or fungal infections of the esophagus. **Upper endoscopy** allows the evaluation of the upper intestine, including the esophagus, stomach, and first portion of the duodenum, using a thin flexible endoscope passed through the mouth. As with colonoscopy, most physicians will provide sedation for patients undergoing upper endoscopy.

Other organs of the body are occasionally involved in the process of inflammatory bowel disease. Liver or bile duct inflammation, although uncommon, can occur in patients with ulcerative colitis or Crohn's disease. Specific diagnosis of this condition may involve a **liver biopsy** obtained by passing a small needle through the side of the abdomen after injection of a local anesthesia. Some physicians may request CT scan or ultrasound-guided biopsy of the liver especially when specific areas of the liver are abnormal. It is possible to visualize the bile ducts connecting to and within the liver using an endoscopic procedure known as **endoscopic retrograde cholangiopancreatography (ERCP),** or by passing a needle through the skin into the bile duct and injecting contrast under radiologic guidance. Fortunately, severe liver disease is uncommon in inflammatory bowel disease and these tests are not often needed.

Preparing for Diagnostic Tests

Diagnostic tests for inflammatory bowel disease can be a time-consuming and sometimes uncomfortable experience. Since each person with IBD is different, your physician will choose only the tests that you need, depending on your symptoms. It is important for you to understand what your physician expects to learn from each of these tests, and how that information may change the treatment of your IBD. Knowing the benefits of the information obtained from a particular test may help alleviate your concerns about discomfort or exposure to radiation, if any during the test, as well as your concern about the cost of the test. Frequent x-rays and endoscopic examinations are neither advisable nor necessary; if your physician orders them, it is not unreasonable for you to ask if the x-ray or endoscopy is essential and why. Ask your physician how your treatment will change as a result of undergoing these studies. It is your physician's job to help you understand the reason for administering each test and the preparation needed for it.

Frequent x-rays and endoscopic examinations are neither advisable nor necessary.

Physicians are becoming increasingly sensitive to your right to receive accurate and complete information about the diagnosis and treatment of your medical condition. Since each test may have associated minor and occasionally major complications, your physician may ask you to sign a consent form indicating that you understand and agree to the procedure. Of the many rights you have, one of the most important is your right to receive accurate and complete information about medical testing.

Bowel Preparations

In order for your doctor to have a clear view during a sigmoidoscopy, colonoscopy or barium enema study, your colon must be completely free of stool prior to the examination. Therefore, you must carefully and accurately follow the special instructions regarding diet, laxatives and, at times, enemas prior to these procedures.

Before a barium enema or colonoscopy, you may be asked to follow a clear liquid diet for one to two days. Clear liquids are those fluids that you can see through and include tea, apple juice, cranberry juice, soda and water, and foods such as clear broth or clear gelatin (See Chapter 16). Laxatives may be prescribed before your tests. These can be tablets such as Dulcolax,® or liquids such as magnesium citrate. If you are experiencing severe diarrhea, significant abdominal tenderness, or cramps, you should inform your physician, since strong laxatives will most likely be omitted from your preparation.

The bowel preparation for a barium enema x-ray will likely include enemas. Using proper technique when taking or giving an enema is vitally important to obtaining a clean bowel. It is best to lie on your left side because this postion uses the normal bowel configuration and gravity to assist in the passage of enema fluid through the rectum and into the left side of of the colon. Gently insert the tip of the lubricated enema tube through the anus and direct it slowly toward the naval for about one and one-half inches. Then redirect the tube so it is pointing toward the base of your spine, and cautiously insert it a few more inches. This technique follows the normal contours of the rectum and will avoid injury to the rectal lining. Hold or suspend the enema bag just above your right hip and allow the contents to flow slowly into the colon. If the fluid is allowed to run in too rapidly, it may stimulate the rectum to expel the fluid prematurely. Elevating the buttocks on a pillow may help in retaining more of the fluid.

Prior to a colonoscopy, some physicians will order a preparation using a large volume laxative (Golytley® or Co-Lyte®). You will need to drink approximately one gallon of this salty tasting liquid, which will induce diarrhea and thus cleanse the bowel. The preparation requires that you drink

approximately one glass of solution every 10 minutes for two to three hours. Some patients prefer to mix the liquid with a sugar-free lemonade or Kool-Aid to enhance the taste of the preparation. Other tricks include drinking the liquid on ice or drinking it through a straw. It will take approximately three hours for all the liquid to pass through your bowel. Of course, it is important to make sure you always have access to a bathroom during this preparation, since it is intended to induce diarrhea.

Sigmoidoscopy

Preparation for a sigmoidoscopy usually includes one or two enemas taken about an hour or two before the procedure. Some physicians may ask that you fast for four to six hours before a sigmoidoscopy, but this is not always necessary. You may take your regular medication unless otherwise instructed by your doctor. Most physicians prefer not to give sedative medications for a sigmoidoscopy, and they are usually unnecessary anyway.

You may begin to note some abdominal pressure as the sigmoidoscope is advanced through the lower bowel.

You will be asked to lie on a table on your left side with your knees flexed. Sometimes a special table is used which can be adjusted so you will be lying in a knee-to-chest or jack-knife position. Your body will be draped with a sheet so that only your buttocks are exposed for the examination. Your doctor will first examine your rectum with a gloved finger and will then insert the sigmoidoscope. You may feel a mild sensation of needing to move your bowels. Small amounts of air are generally injected through the sigmoidoscope during the procedure to help to distend the rectum and colon for better visualization. This may cause an uncomfortable sensation of cramping or bloating. You may begin to note some abdominal pressure as the sigmoidoscope is advanced through the lower bowel. You will feel discomfort but you should not feel pain. If you do experience any pain during the procedure, be sure to let your doctor know immediately. The procedure itself takes only about 5 to 10 minutes.

During the examination, try to relax your abdominal muscles to prevent any discomfort caused by muscle tension. Regular rhythmic breathing may help you to do this. After the procedure, some air may remain in the bowel which will need to be expelled along with any remaining enema liquid. A visit to the bathroom after this procedure will make you more comfortable before going home.

Colonoscopy

When preparing for a colonoscopy, it is advisable to stop taking any aspirin products, bulking agents, and iron preparations for about one week before the examination. Aspirin increases the risk of bleeding if biopsies are required. Bulking agents like Metamucil® make cleansing the bowel more difficult. Iron preparations will sometimes adhere to the lining of the colon making these areas difficult to visualize.

Before the colonoscopy and after the doctor has explained the procedure and answered all your questions, you will be asked to sign a consent form. Be sure to inform your doctor or nurse if you are allergic to any drugs or to adhesive tape. You may also be asked to remove any dentures or contact lenses. You will be asked to lie on your left side and sedative medications will be given by intravenous or intramuscular injection.

Since the colon has no surface nerve endings, biopsies are painless.

After you have been adequately sedated, the doctor will examine your rectum with a gloved finger, and will insert the flexible colonoscope gently into your rectum. The physician will advance the tube slowly through the colon, examining the lining thoroughly. You may feel some abdominal cramping caused by the air which is injected into the colon through the colonoscope, and by the movement of the colonoscope when it is advanced around turns in the colon. Occasionally during the examination, the nurse may apply pressure with her hands to your abdomen to help with the passage of the instrument. You may also be asked to change positions. Infrequently, fluoroscopy (x-ray equipment) may be used to define the location of the colonoscope within the bowel. Biopsies may be taken during the colonoscopy for microscopic examination. Since the colon has no surface nerve endings, these biopsies are painless. The colonoscopic examination takes from 20 minutes to one hour. After the procedure, you will be transferred to another room to sleep or rest until the effect of the medication partially wears off. You may feel some bloating from the air which remains in the colon. As the air is expelled, your abdomen will become more comfortable.

Since you will have received medications or sedation that may have a prolonged effect and may interfere with your ability to drive or operate heavy machinery, it is important that you make arrangements for someone to drive you home the day of the examination.

Occasionally, local irritation may occur at the site used for injecting the sedatives. You can use warm compresses on this area, if necessary. If you notice excessive pain, redness, or warmth at the injection site, be sure to notify your physician. You should also report any fever, abdominal pain, or rectal bleeding. If biopsies were performed, your doctor may ask you to avoid aspirin or other arthritis-type medications for up to 10 days after the procedure, since these medications tend to aggravate bleeding.

Upper Gastrointestinal Endoscopy

In order for the physician to have clear view of your upper digestive tract, your stomach must be completely empty. This generally requires that you fast for at least 8 to 12 hours before examination. Avoid any lozenges, hard candy, and antacids that coat and discolor the lining of the esophagus and stomach, and interfere with the accuracy of the examination. You should check with your doctor about whether to take your usual medications.

As with a colonoscopy, you will be asked to sign a consent form to authorize your doctor to perform this examination. You should ask all your questions about the procedure before you are sedated. All dentures and contact lenses must be removed prior to the start of the examination. The physician may spray the back of your throat with an anesthetic to numb the throat and prevent gagging. If necessary, sedative medications will be given by injection. You will be asked to turn on your left side and a small plastic mouthpiece will be placed between your teeth. When you are relaxed, your physician will place the endoscopic tube through the mouthpiece into the back of your mouth and ask you to swallow. It is normal to feel a strong gagging reflex, but this will pass. A bloating sensation may occur as air is introduced through the endoscope to allow visualization of the stomach. Belching is common. During the procedure, a nurse will suction saliva from your mouth and throat. Because breathing occurs through the trachea, upper endoscopy will not interfere with your ability to breathe. As with colonoscopy or sigmoidoscopy, biopsies may be taken for microscopic examination.

Like upper endoscopy, an ERCP is performed by passing an endoscope through your mouth into your esophagus, stomach, and duodenum. Once the endoscope is in the duodenum, you will be asked to lie nearly flat on your stomach with your left hand placed off to the side. This procedure is performed with a special endoscope and x-rays are needed to provide pictures of the bile ducts.

An endoscopy lasts about 15 to 30 minutes and an ERCP takes approximately one hour. After the endoscopy is completed, you will be moved to another room to rest until the effect of the medication partially wears off. Unless your doctor or nurse indicates otherwise, you will be able to resume eating about four to six hours after the procedure. As with a colonoscopy, because of the sedating effects of the medicine you should plan to have someone drive you home the day of the procedure.

You may notice a scratchy throat following the procedure. This can be relieved by using lozenges, gargles, or by drinking soothing beverages such as warm tea. If the symptoms persist over 24 hours or worsen, you should notify your doctor. You should also notify your physician if you have any fever, chest or abdominal pain, or passage of bloody or black stools.

Summary

When diagnostic testing is performed under the guidance of a skilled physician, valuable information can be obtained about your medical condition. Understanding the nature and purpose of tests will help minimize your stress, discomfort, and anxiety. A properly performed diagnostic evaluation can be a valuable tool to define your disease and plan appropriate treatment.

Knowing What to Expect: Symptoms and Extent of Disease

3

Knowing what to expect from an illness usually helps people to cope better and stay in control. This is true of IBD and most chronic conditions. As a general rule, the symptoms of both Crohn's disease and ulcerative colitis, as well as the response to medical treatment and the possible complications, will vary with the part of the intestinal tract that is inflamed. This is why it is very important to know just which part or parts of intestine are involved. This chapter will describe the symptoms you might expect from both Crohn's disease and ulcerative colitis, depending upon the location and extent of inflammation.

The symptoms of both Crohn's disease and ulcerative colitis, as well as the response to medical treatment and the possible complications, will vary with the part of the intestinal tract that is inflamed.

Crohn's Disease: Where Is My Disease?

Ileitis or Ileocolitis
Crohn's disease most commonly involves the lower one or two feet of the ileum, the lower third of the small intestine, often in combination with the cecum, the first part of the colon containing the appendix (See diagram). Inflammation caused by Crohn's disease is called **ileitis** if it involves only the ileum and **ileocolitis** if it involves both ileum and cecum. About half of all patients with Crohn's disease first come to the physician with ileocolitis.

Ileitis and ileocolitis, like Crohn's disease elsewhere, starts as small focal areas of inflammation in the inner lining of the bowel, or mucosa. Small **apthous ulcers** begin to form on top of the inflammation. These small sores in the mucosa can be present for two or three years without causing bowel symptoms. For example, some teenagers who have not yet reached puberty will eat normally, will not have any intestinal symptoms, but will have delayed growth for one or two years before any obvious symptoms of Crohn's disease appear. Most recently, we have learned that this early phase, characterized by aphthous ulcers, can be present without any obvious symptoms. Frequently, these aphthous ulcers can be seen by colonoscopy following resection of the terminal ileum and reconnection of the ileum to the colon. This phenomenon has been observed in the **proximal** (upper) ileum in about 80 percent of patients one year after surgery. These individuals may have no symptoms for several years, even though small ulcers are present.

What process causes the uncomfortable symptoms of ileocolitis? With time the sores or ulcerations become more numerous, larger, and deeper. (These same aphthous ulcerations are found occasionally in the mouths of people experiencing a flare-up of Crohn's disease.) The wall of the ileum then becomes swollen and thickened. The area may resemble a cobblestone street with bumps and valleys. This process both narrows and irritates this part of the intestine. The lumen, or hollow part of the ileum, is normally about one or two inches wide and is easily stretched. In Crohn's disease, the ileum becomes rigid and narrow (somewhat like a garden hose) and easily goes into spasm. At times, the lumen may narrow to the width of a pencil or even a string during spasm. It is this narrowed or cobblestoned appearance that first suggests the presence of Crohn's disease to the radiologist and gastroenterologist.

What Symptoms to Expect from Ileitis or Ileocolitis

If you have ileitis or ileocolitis, you may notice a cramping or dull pain in the right lower part of the abdomen about 60 to 90 minutes after a meal. This discomfort usually lasts for a few minutes and may feel like a "gas" pain. It may come and go, getting worse, then better, then worse again. At times, the pain is so severe that you double over, pull up your knees, bite your lip or even cry out in discomfort. At times, the pain will be felt in the middle of the abdomen, around the belly-button, because of stretching or distension of the small intestine above the inflamed area. To avoid this pain, some people eat less, lose weight, and do not even realize they are avoiding eating. Abdominal pain is so common in this form of Crohn's disease that about two-thirds of patients first come to the doctor complaining of pain. Weight loss at the time of diagnosis is also extremely common in people with ileocolitis: 10 percent of patients will have lost over one fifth of their body weight.

Abdominal pain is so common in Crohn's disease that about two-thirds of patients first come to the doctor complaining of pain.

What Your Doctor Finds at Examination

When first examined by the physician, only half of those with ileitis or ileocolitis have any tenderness or feeling of fullness in the abdomen. The other half have no localizing signs on physical examination. For this reason, the physician needs to have a high degree of suspicion to even consider the diagnosis of Crohn's disease when examining a patient with abdominal pain. This may explain why some people with ileitis or ileocolitis may go for several years without a diagnosis until other symptoms make their appearance.

Another reason for the delay in diagnosis may be the absence of diarrhea. Only one of five patients with ileitis has diarrhea as a chief complaint when the diagnosis is first made. Why? Because, even though the inflamed ileum may squirt intestinal contents quickly through into the colon, the remaining five or six feet of healthy colon can store the liquid contents for many hours. Since much of this extra fluid may be reabsorbed through the wall of the colon, the person with ileitis may have one formed bowel movement a day or perhaps two or three soft stools, not enough to alert the physician to the presence of Crohn's disease.

Occasionally problems such as fever, joint pains, or painful, tender bumps on the skin may be the symptoms that bring people with ileitis or ileocolitis to the physician for the first time. Because the intestinal symptoms may not be obvious, some patients, especially adolescents, may go four to six months without a specific diagnosis.

Eventually, most people with ileitis or ileocolitis begin to notice some diarrhea. In addition, the ulcerations in the ileum or right colon may weep small amounts of blood. This blood is usually hidden in the stool **(occult blood)** and is not visible on the toilet paper. Occult blood can be detected with a chemical test of the stool, such as a Hemoccult® test. This subtle blood loss may go on for months, causing iron deficiency and anemia, weakness, fatigue, and a pale skin color.

Jejunoileitis

The jejunum is the upper half of the small intestine starting just after the duodenum, which connects to the stomach. **Jejunoileitis** is the term used to describe Crohn's disease involving several "skip" areas in the small bowel. About 20 to 30 percent of those with Crohn's disease have this rather widespread problem. Their symptoms of abdominal pain and cramps start soon after meals and may be accompanied by nausea and loss of appetite if the duodenum is also inflamed. Because of the pain and loss of appetite, weight loss may be prominent. Since the jejunum is the part of the intestine where most food is absorbed by the body, inflammation in this area causes malabsorption, weight loss, and foul-smelling stools.

Crohn's Colitis

It is now known that one doesn't have to have ileitis to have Crohn's disease. **Colitis** (disease in the colon alone) is the main problem for one of five patients with Crohn's disease. Sometimes it is difficult for the gastroenterologist to tell if a patient has Crohn's colitis or ulcerative colitis because the symptoms are so similar. Even after surgery about 5 to 10 percent of patients may still be listed as "indeterminate."

People with Crohn's colitis almost always have diarrhea at some point in their illness. Rectal bleeding and disease around the anus are also more common than in ileitis or jejunoileitis. Some extra-intestinal problems,

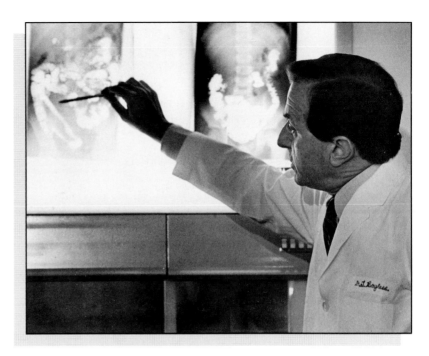

A gastroenterologist observes the x-rays of a patient with Crohn's disease.

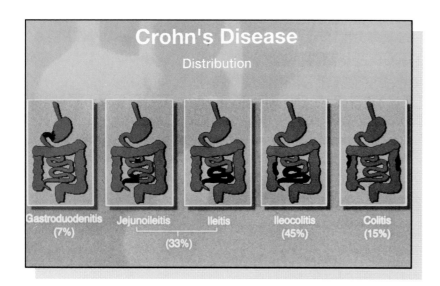

Locations of Crohn's disease in the intestine.

such as skin lesions and joint pains, also seem to be more common with Crohn's colitis (See below).

Other complications of Crohn's colitis such as severe bleeding, perforations or abscesses usually occur in the first five years of disease and usually require surgery. Obstruction occurs occasionally in the colon, but much less often than in the small intestine; surgery is not commonly needed for colon obstruction. Although medical treatment is often successful in avoiding removal of the colon, people with extensive Crohn's colitis are at a somewhat increased risk of developing colon cancer after approximately 10 to 15 years of disease.

Extra-intestinal Manifestations and Crohn's Disease

Most of the "extra-intestinal" signs and symptoms of Crohn's disease are related to disease activity and usually decrease when the intestinal inflammation is treated medically. Joint problems occur in about 5 to 10 percent of people with Crohn's disease and include pain and swelling in the knees, hips, ankles or wrists. Some people develop low back pain caused by inflammation of the sacroiliac joints **(sacroileitis)**, and experience morning stiffness. Eye problems, such as **iritis** or **uveitis** cause blurred vision, redness or eye pain; these are more common with colonic disease, occurring in 1 of 25 patients with Crohn's colitis or ileocolitis. Serious skin disorders, such as **erythema nodosum** (painful red swellings on the shins) or **pyoderma gangrenosum** (painful, deep ulcerations on the legs or forearms) are also more common in patients with Crohn's colitis. Erythema nodosum does heal when bowel symptoms are controlled medically: pyoderma gangrenosum is more unpredictable. Apthous ulcers in the mouth may recur together with a flare-up of the intestinal inflammation.

Complications Requiring Surgery

As you will read elsewhere in this book, most episodes of Crohn's disease can be controlled using a variety of treatments (medical and surgical), either alone or in combination. (See Chapter 5 for an explanation of IBD medications and their use.) However, even in patients with easily controlled ileitis or ileocolitis, scarring and narrowing of the lower ileum seems to proceed both with and without symptoms. In about 6 of every 10 patients, the ileum becomes so narrowed after 8 or 10 years of disease that severe cramps begin soon after meals. These new symptoms may be quite severe if the bowel becomes partially obstructed. If this happens, you will be able to recognize that your symptoms have changed. You may avoid eating or vomit after a meal, and may lose a considerable amount of weight. Family and friends may notice loud bowel sounds caused by the partial obstruction. Repeat small bowel x-rays or CT scans will usually confirm that the ileum is so scarred and narrowed that the bowel above it has begun to dilate. This may be an ideal time to consider resection of the lower ileum and part of the right colon. The recurrence rate of Crohn's disease after such a limited resection is lowest if the length of bowel removed is short, if there are no complications other than obstruction, and if the Crohn's disease isn't very active. More research is needed to decide on the best course of medical treatment to prevent recurrent disease after bowel resection. At present, there are no medications that can accomplish this.

Fissures (cracks), fistulas (abnormal openings), and abscesses (pockets of infections) around the rectum, referred to as **perirectal** or **perianal** disease, are a frequent complication of Crohn's disease. If a fissure or fistula causes a lot of pain, some degree of infection, such as a small localized abscess, is often suspected. An abscess will sometimes drain spontaneously with warm baths or medications, but can be quickly and easily drained surgically. Most people with Crohn's disease who have perirectal disease are only bothered occasionally. However, in some people this becomes the main focus of their medical problem, requiring special medications and occasionally, surgery. At times, a flare-up of the perirectal disease will be a signal that the intestinal problem is again active or about to become active.

Ulcerative Colitis: Degrees of Inflammation

The term ulcerative colitis means that there is a characteristic inflammatory process going on in the colon, or large intestine. The word colitis itself means inflammation of the colon, and the degree of inflammation can vary from mild to severe. Since ulcerative colitis *always* involves the rectal segment of the colon, this inflammation can easily be seen by the physician who looks at it with an instrument called a sigmoidoscope. The degrees of inflammation seen through the sigmoidoscope can be classified in the following way:

1. **Mild Inflammation:**
   The lining of the rectum looks normal or a little red (**erythematous**); obviously, a diagnosis of ulcerative colitis cannot be made by these findings alone. The physician will gently rub the mucosal surface with a cotton swab. Even this mild stroking can cause the mucosal surface to bleed. Easy bleeding on the mucosal surface is called **friability;** it means that mild inflammation, suggestive of ulcerative colitis, is present.
2. **Moderate Inflammation:**
   Spots of blood are apparent even without rubbing. The spots actually

identify the sites of tiny ulcers covering the mucosal surface. Often the lining of the rectum is also covered with patches of mucus; if the mucus has a yellowish or greenish tint, this indicates the presence of pus or exudate. The combination of mucus and pus is often referred to as **muco-pus.**

3. **Moderate to Severe Inflammation:** Blood is seen immediately upon the introduction of the sigmoidoscope, whether lying free within the rectum or oozing when the instrument touches the mucosal surface. The tiny ulcerations will have merged so that the entire surface bleeds and has a raw or eroded look. The surface also appears bumpy or pock-marked, the way the skin looks in measles or chicken-pox. This is called **granularity** and is caused by the varying degrees of inflammatory activity. The amount of muco-pus varies; in some cases, it dominates the appearance while in others the bleeding is more evident.

4. **Severe Inflammation:** Any resemblance to normal rectal mucosa has disappeared. The sigmoidoscope confronts liquid blood and pus, which make it difficult to examine the underlying mucosa. Furthermore, the lumen of the rectum may be narrowed by the underlying disease encroaching from all sides.

The physician may also see mounds of tissue of various shapes at any of the above stages of inflammation. These are called **pseudopolyps,** tissues that remain intact after the surrounding inflammatory tissue has subsided, eroded, or sloughed. They are not *true* polyps and do not mean that there is any premalignant change in the bowel surface. Occasionally, however, the physician will take a **biopsy** (tissue sample) to be sure that they are not true polyps.

Where Is My Disease?

Since ulcerative colitis always involves the rectum—(unlike Crohn's disease which often does not), the diagnosis is relatively easy to make. When a person has rectal bleeding, the physician need only examine the rectum with a sigmoidoscope to see the inflammation. After examining tissue taken during biopsies, the pathologist will usually report that the findings are "consistent with a diagnosis of ulcerative colitis." Those findings are not *specific* and therefore not absolutely diagnostic of ulcerative colitis. The main reason for taking the biopsy is to differentiate the ulcerative colitis from other types of colitis, particularly Crohn's disease involving the rectum and infectious types of colitis caused by bacteria and parasites.

For some people with the disease, perhaps about half, ulcerative colitis involves only the rectal segment and is called **ulcerative proctitis.** In fact, in about 75 to 90 percent of those with ulcerative proctitis, the inflammation remains confined to the rectum throughout life, no matter how severe the disease might become locally. It is important for the physisian to determine whether the disease is truly proctitis (i.e. confined to the rectum) and not more extensive. Since the conventional rigid sigmoidoscope can easily reach 8 to 12 inches beyond the anal margin, the entire rectum and some of the sigmoid colon can easily be inspected. If the physician sees moderate inflammation at this level, it is then impossible to tell how far upward the inflammation extends, and whether it is proctitis or colitis (involving the colon and rectum.) To determine where inflammation ends and normal-appearing tissue begins, the physician uses a 35 cm or 60 cm flexible sigmoidoscope in an effort to determine the true extent of disease.

Some people with ulcerative colitis have disease involving the next segment of colon, the sigmoid colon, in conjunction with the upper part of the rectum. This is called **proctosigmoiditis.** Just as with proctitis, the inflammation is likely to remain confined to that segment even though symptoms may worsen. Nevertheless, there is a possibility that the disease will spread further up the length of colon.

The next classification of ulcerative colitis is called **distal** or **left-sided colitis.** In left-sided colitis, there may be continuous inflammation from rectum to descending colon, rectum to splenic flexure, and even from rectum to transverse colon. As in all distributions of ulcerative colitis, the rectum is involved, and the inflammation is continuous up to the point where normal tissue begins.

A fourth classification is extensive or **universal ulcerative colitis,** in which inflammation extends up to the mid-transverse colon and beyond, usually all the way to the cecum, the last part of the colon before it joins the small intestine. Occasionally even the end of the small intestine, the terminal ileum may be inflamed for a very short distance. Although involvement of the terminal ileum is far more characteristic of Crohn's disease, in those few cases of so-called "**backwash ileitis**" caused by ulcerative colitis, the inflammation actually *looks* like ulcerative colitis and not like Crohn's disease. In most cases of ulcerative colitis, the more intestine that is involved, the more severe the symptoms will be and the worse the prognosis.

What Symptoms Will I Have?

The symptoms of ulcerative colitis vary with the extent of the disease and the speed of its onset. With proctitis, it is possible to pass blood through the rectum and nothing more. Unlike

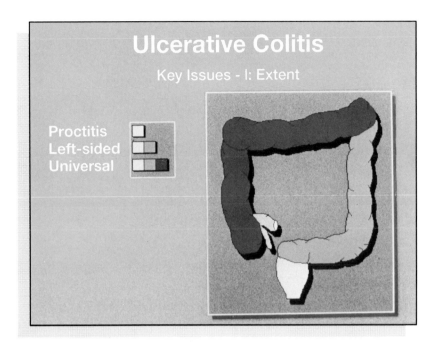

Distribution of types of ulcerative colitis.

blood from hemorrhoids or a rectal fissure, the blood from ulcerative proctitis is less likely to be seen on the toilet paper and more likely to be found in the toilet bowl. If the disease involves only an inch or two of the rectum, the stool may remain normally formed and the blood will coat the outer surface. If it involves several inches, more often the blood will be passed into the bowl without stool, probably mixed with mucus and/or pus. If blood is accompanied by stool, the stool often will be loose.

The more extensive the inflamed surface of bowel, the less opportunity there is for water or liquid stool to be reabsorbed.

With more extensive disease there is true diarrhea, usually bloody diarrhea. The more extensive the inflamed surface of bowel, the less opportunity there is for water or liquid stool passing through the colon to be reabsorbed; also, more extensive inflammation causes a larger volume of mucus, pus and blood, making it even less likely that you will have a formed stool. Only in ulcerative proctitis and proctosigmoiditis is it possible to pass blood and mucus and then, afterwards, a formed stool. This is because the stool forms in the normal colon above the inflamed rectal and sigmoid segments. It is held there, usually by a spasm in the inflamed rectum, causing a feeling of constipation. Once the blood and mucus have passed and the spasm has relaxed, the formed stool can be passed.

Another common symptom is the sense of bowel urgency and rectal discomfort called **tenesmus.** This can be interpreted as the bowel's being unable to rest. Even with proctitis, the tenesmus can be a problem. However, some people with proctitis pass blood and/or pus without discomfort. Even when there is more extensive disease, pain as such is not an outstanding symptom. Cramps and urgency are common symptoms in proctosigmoiditis, although some people report severe abdominal pain on the left side. In general, pain is far more common in Crohn's disease than in ulcerative colitis.

How Does Ulcerative Colitis Begin?

More often than not, the onset of ulcerative colitis is slow and passage of blood and loosening of the stool are the initial symptoms. Rarely, the disease begins rapidly, with cramps and bloody diarrhea following an infectious illness such as a flu, a course of antibiotics, or an emotional tragedy such as loss of a dear one or a depression. (This does not mean that emotional factors caused the disease, rather that they may have triggered its onset.) Recently, quitting smoking has been identified as a factor in triggering flare-ups of ulcerative colitis. However, just as often, the disease begins without the presence of any of these factors!

In general, the symptoms you will feel are determined by how much of the colon is diseased and by how quickly the inflammation has spread. If no diagnosis is made and no treatment begun, the disease could progress to include the following:

1. Dehydration as a result of loss of water in the diarrhea.
2. Fever when the inflammatory process is advanced.
3. Extraintestinal manifestations, including arthritis (of medium sized joints), uveitis (eye inflammation) and skin lesions, such as erythema nodosum and pyoderma gangrenosum.

4. Progressively severe bleeding causing anemia and occasionally hemorrhage requiring blood transfusions.
5. Loss of protein into the bowel with resulting loss of blood proteins and edema (swelling).
6. Progressive severity of the inflammation with sloughing of the bowel lining and possible perforation.
7. Toxic megacolon, or dilation of the colon in respose to the spread of the inflammatory process throughout the bowel wall. The development of toxic megacolon requires urgent and intensive treatment to reverse its course and prevent perforation of the colon.

Fortunately, *all* of these can be alleviated with the proper medical treatment. Ulcerative colitis, regardless of extent, is not a disease that lends itself to spontaneous remission. There are exceptions to this, and many people avoid seeing the physician because of the mildness of symptoms and the hope and expectation that they will disappear. In most cases however, the sooner the diagnosis and recognition of complications, the sooner appropriate medical therapy can begin. The early establishment of a partnership between you and your gastroenterologist increases the chances that remission will be achieved and maintained. (Chapter 5 contains a full explanation of the medications currently used to control the symptoms of ulcerative colitis.)

Knowing What to Expect from Treatment

With the proper timing and choice of medications, it is possible to predict the outcome of ulcerative colitis. The symptoms of ulcerative proctitis and most proctosigmoiditis can be controlled and can remain in remission most of the time. In more extensive disease, worsening of symptoms is likely to occur, but renewed medical treatment will usually lead to another remission. Most recurrences of ulcerative colitis occur in the first 10 years of disease. After that, recurrences become less frequent but the risk of cancer of the colon increases. This risk is a product of the greater extent of disease and its duration. Fortunately, periodic examination of the colon with the colonoscope as well as removal of tissue (biopsy) can reveal early precancerous lesions called **dysplasia.** If dysplasia is found, removal of the colon **(colectomy)** is usually recommended. This operation both removes the threat of cancer *and* cures the ulcerative colitis. Chapters 6 and 7 contain information about ileostomies and about the new operations that do not require an ileostomy appliance.

Most recurrences of ulcerative colitis occur in the first 10 years of disease.

For people with ulcerative colitis, particularly those with left-sided and universal disease who have responded successfully to the use of medications, compliance becomes an important issue. When you are feeling well, it is normal to want to avoid all reminders of previous illness and, in doing so, avoid the physician and the regular colonoscopies that are a part of regular follow-up of the disease. However, experience has shown that people who come in for regular follow-up, including colonoscopy with biopsy, and keep in regular touch with their physicians, have a better prognosis and can prevent the occasional cancer that arises after long-term extensive disease.

What's the Worst Thing That Can Happen to Me?

4

Fears about Losing Control

One of the most embarrassing possibilities and one of the biggest fears for someone with diarrhea is the loss of bowel control. Unfortunately, diarrhea and urgency are common symptoms of both ulcerative colitis and Crohn's disease. This leads many people to seek out the nearest bathroom in any new environment. They know every clean restroom along a highway or along their daily route, and become anxious anytime there is a crowd with limited toilet facilities. Some people are afraid to travel away from home and can even become reclusive if these fears are overwhelming.

Fortunately, most people with IBD are able to adapt to the demands of diarrhea. Of course, there may be more problems when the illness is active, but in most situations there are ways to deal with the symptoms of diarrhea and urgency. The most important of these is to gain control over the inflammation with a regular schedule of medications. Bowel activity is directly related to food intake; therefore, it may be best to avoid eating if you have a special engagement, at least until you are within reach of a restroom. Highly spicy or greasy foods tend to induce more bowel movements and should be avoided along with any food that tends to stimulate bowel activity (e.g. caffeine, gassy vegetables, or fruits). Antidiarrheal medications can reduce frequency but may aggravate gas or cramping. Adequate cleansing around the anal area (with moistened towelettes or sitz baths) will reduce any irritiation. Finally, you may feel more relaxed if you wear a disposable pad or undergarment, or carry a spare pair of underpants.

Individuals with stomas have special concerns about loss of control and leakage. Again, experience is the best teacher and most people will develop their own system to handle each situation. It is rare for a stoma to cause problems once you have become adjusted to it. Avoiding eating at certain times (e.g. before physical activity, sex, etc.) will minimize worries about leakage and overfilling of the ostomy bag. If there are continued problems, a discussion with an experienced enterostomal therapist or surgeon should identify the cause and produce a solution.

Sexual function may be a concern for a variety of reasons: loss of bowel control, exposure of scars or an ostomy appliance, fear of inadequacy, etc. We all must realize that intimate relations require openess and honesty between couples; a frank discussion of your fears with your partner is essential. Take things gradually until you learn each other's "systems" and communicate as you proceed. Communication, honesty, and ingenuity will go a long way toward satisfying your physical and emotional needs and those of your partner.

People with any chronic illness worry that their illness will prevent them from engaging in sports or other physical activities. Of course, during an acute episode of IBD, it may be necessary to halt intensive physical activity temporarily. However, most people are able to resume their activity schedule once symptoms improve. As we have learned from the athletes featured elsewhere in this book, there are very few ultimate restrictions caused by IBD (See Chapter 18).

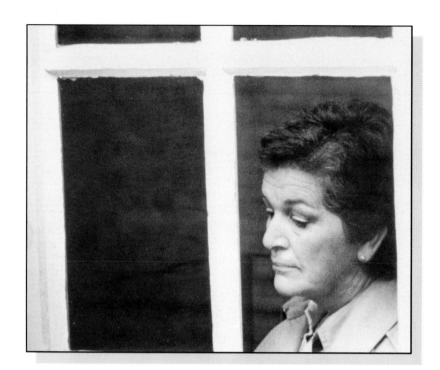

Will I Need to Have Surgery?

One of the biggest worries for a person with IBD is about the need for surgery. Some people fear the pain associated with an operation, the loss of control while under anesthesia, or the possibility that they will not wake-up after the operation. Others fear they will be disfigured by the surgical scars. Underlying these fears is often the dread of ostomy surgery and the trauma to body image and self-esteem introduced by that operation.

To address these very real concerns, it is necessary to look first at why operations are performed for IBD and how often they are necessary. In ulcerative colitis, surgery is necessary when an attack is so severe that the colon is at risk of perforating, a condition known as toxic megacolon. Fortunately, this is now a rare event and occurs in less than 5 percent of all patients. Other indications for surgery include severe bleeding, the failure to respond to medical treatment, or the development of cancer. In general, about one in four or five people with ulcerative colitis ever needs surgery.

In Crohn's disease, surgery is needed for complications that will not improve with medication, such as obstruction, abscess, bleeding, or perforation. An operation may also be recommended if there is no improvement of symptoms with medication or if medications cause serious side effects. Unfortunately, operations are more common in Crohn's disease; about two-thirds to three-quarters of people need surgery at some time during their lives.

Only about half of those who undergo an operation for Crohn's disease will need additional surgery for recurrent disease.

When operations are necessary, the result is most often a return to good health. In the case of ulcerative colitis, this means a return to health *and* a cure for the disease. Although surgery does not cure Crohn's disease, it often alleviates serious problems and results in significant improvement. Only about half of those who undergo an operation for Crohn's disease will need additional surgery for recurrent disease. Multiple operations throughout life are the exception rather than the rule.

Another misconception about IBD surgery is that an ostomy is necessary in most situations. Again, the need for a stoma has become the exception rather than the rule. In ulcerative colitis, it is now possible to remove the colon and maintain continuity of the intestine so that there is no need for a permanent ileostomy. Surgery for Crohn's disease can usually be accomplished without the need for a stoma. By far, the most common operation in Crohn's disease is resection of a diseased segment of intestine with reconnection (anastomosis) of the two ends. Only in severe cases of Crohn's colitis is a permanent ileostomy necessary; a temporary ileostomy is sometimes required for several months after emergency surgery for a bowel perforation or abscess. You can be assured that in the great majority of situations, life returns to normal after an operation. Even after ostomy surgery, a return to full health can be expected.

Fears about Dying

Am I going to die? Is my spouse/child/parent going to die? This question is often never *actually* asked by people with IBD or their loved ones; but it is there nonetheless, stimulated by the development of frightening symptoms like bleeding, persistent diarrhea, uncontrolled weight loss, or worsening abdominal pain. Ironically, this fear often prevents people from discussing their symptoms with family members, let alone

What Do We Worry About? National Survey Reveals Fears and Concerns of People with IBD

People with IBD readily tell their doctors about bowel symptoms but may not disclose the deep-seated worries that trouble them. Likewise, few investigators have researched the specific fears and concerns of people with IBD; the few published studies in existence have used a fixed list of questions generated by physicians, rather than asking open-ended questions to get at what is really on patients' minds.

In a recently published national study of 997 people, all members of the Crohn's & Colitis Foundation of America, **Dr. Douglas A. Drossman** and co-workers from the University of North Carolina used a new self-report measure they call the Rating Form of Inflammatory Bowel Disease Patient Concerns (RFIPC). This scale, constructed after interviewing IBD patients on videotape, lists the 25 fears and concerns they mentioned most often and includes many hard-to-discuss items such as fears about sexual intimacy, loss of control, pain and suffering, feeling alone, and being able to acheive full potential.

The number-one concern for people with either form of IBD was the uncertainty caused by having the disease, followed closely by worries about the side effects of medications, having enough energy to go about daily activities, and having surgery, particularly ostomy surgery. People with Crohn's disease worried more about their energy level, being a burden on others, reaching their full potential, having pain, and dealing with financial difficulties caused by the disease. Those with ulcerative colitis worried more about developing cancer.

(Continued on next page)

(Continued from previous page)

The researchers found that those with the greatest number of IBD-related fears and concerns had a poorer quality of life (that is, ability to function, sense of general well-being, and perception of health). As might be expected, they also found that younger patients were more concerned with the impact of the disease on their future and about sexual intimacy. Dr. Drossman cautions that because all those surveyed are members of the CCFA and derive the added benefit of social support and education, they may cope better and have fewer worries than others with the disease.

Learning about the fears and concerns of people with IBD is important to understanding how well we adjust to having these chronic conditions; it's also the first step in designing effective education and support programs to allay these fears.

with the physician, because they fear hearing the worst. Many people even deny the symptoms to themselves, hoping they will go away. Fearing that the symptoms of IBD are actually those of cancer also keeps some individuals from seeking help.

Several careful studies have examined the risk of succumbing to an attack of IBD; others have compared the life expectancy of people with IBD to that of the general public. Despite the fact that Crohn's disease and ulcerative colitis are chronic illnesses that can affect many aspects of health, it is very unlikely that a person will die from an attack of IBD, from surgery, or from any related illness. In fact, most people with IBD live as long as other people their own age; when they die, it is usually from an unrelated cause.

Most people with IBD live as long as other people their own age; when they die, it is usually from an unrelated cause.

Many people have been told about the risk of cancer with ulcerative colitis of long duration (or with longstanding Crohn's disease of the colon.) While there *is* a risk of developing cancer after many decades of disease, with continuing surveillance by the physician, the long-term outlook continues to improve. Even the medications used to treat IBD, in general, have a long record of safety when used appropriately. Overall, despite the disappointment at developing disturbing symptoms and having an unwanted chronic illness, the great majority of people with IBD will survive and live normal lives.

Still, many people are unwilling to voice their concerns to physicians. It is important to do so, and it is important for the physician to be aware of these often unmentioned fears. At times, your doctor may try to maintain an upbeat, positive attitude, ignoring unasked questions and denying some of your fears. It is *always* important to discuss your concerns openly, whether at the time of diagnosis, in the midst of a severe attack, or before surgery. You may find that when they are brought out into the open, your fears are exaggerated or unfounded.

"Disease" Versus "Illness": Living a Normal Life with IBD

"Disease" is the definition of pathology as it affects the body, whereas "illness" is how *you,* as an individual, feel the effects of the disease. Although Crohn's disease and ulcerative colitis are chronic diseases, having one of these diseases, does not mean you will always feel "ill." People with IBD are all individuals, and as individuals they handle each situation differently. Most people with IBD are able to recover from any acute episode of illness and get on with their lives.

As the rest of this book emphasizes, people with IBD can expect to live normally with some accomodation to the demands of illness. Despite the diagnosis of a potentially life-long condition, the burden of taking regular medications, and the occasional need for surgery, most patients are able to lead normal, productive lives. They are, indeed most often "people, not patients!" The great majority of individuals with IBD are able to grow normally, finish school, pursue virtually any occupation, marry and have children. It may take a little longer to achieve these goals, but they *can* be achieved.

Part II

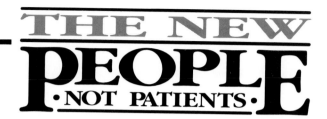

Understanding IBD Treatments

IBD Medications and Their Side Effects

5

Since there is no medical cure for inflammatory bowel disease, the goals of medical treatment are to suppress the inflammatory response, permit healing of tissue, and relieve the symptoms of diarrhea, abdominal pain and fever. As inflammation subsides and symptoms resolve, the person with IBD enters a quiescent phase of illness called a **remission.** This remission may last for a few weeks or for many years. At times the remission is prolonged only if medications are continued; at other times the remission persists even after medications have been discontinued. A remission does not necessarily mean that all active inflammation has subsided, or that the inflamed tissue has healed completely. A remission does mean that you are once again comfortable and able to resume normal activities.

This chapter will focus on the major medications used to treat IBD and will provide information about their use, doses and available preparations, and commonly encountered side effects. The chapter concludes with a discussion of the problem of possible addiction to the medications used to control pain and diarrhea.

Sulfasalazine— Its Use in IBD

Sulfasalazine (often marketed as Azulfidine®) is an effective treatment for mild to moderate episodes of ulcerative colitis. In severe episodes, a corticosteroid preparation administered intravenously is usually needed (See below). After ulcerative colitis has responded to sulfasalazine, it is usually continued in order to prolong the

clinical remission. This recommendation is based on evidence that the risk of a flare-up is significantly lower if the medication is continued.

Sulfasalazine is also effective in treating mild to moderate episodes of Crohn's disease, especially when the colon is involved. Although this medication is less effective in treating Crohn's disease confined to the ileum (ileitis), it is often prescribed initially rather than the more powerful corticosteroid agents. Unlike its usefulness in maintaining a remission in ulcerative colitis, sulfasalazine does not provide this benefit in Crohn's disease. Also, maintenance therapy with sulfasalazine does not prevent recurrences of Crohn's disease after surgical removal of diseased tissue.

Preparations and Doses

Sulfasalazine is available as an oral preparation in several forms: a tablet (500 mg); an enteric-coated tablet (500 mg) that helps prevent upper digestive symptoms; and a suspension for those who have difficulty swallowing a large tablet. The usual dosage is 2–4 grams/day (4–8 tablets). For some people, a dose of 2 grams provides excellent therapy, and there is no need to increase the dose further. Taking sulfasalazine with meals or with a snack helps prevent digestive side effects which can sometimes develop with this medication.

Sulfasalazine contains two active ingredients—a sulfa preparation (sulfapyridine) and an aspirin-like drug (5-aminosalicylic acid or 5-ASA)—which are bonded together. Most of the drug arrives intact in the colon, where bacterial enzymes break the bond that links the two ingredients. The sulfapyridine, which

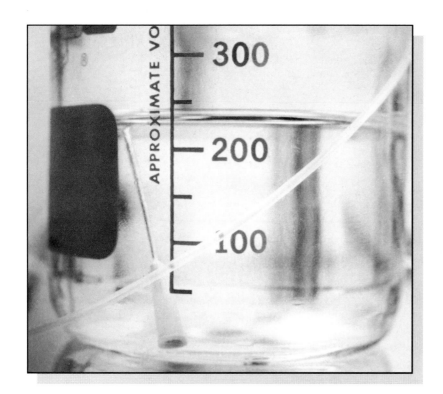

provides no therapeutic benefit, is absorbed into the bloodstream and is responsible for most of the unpleasant and at times serious side effects. The 5-ASA is absorbed only slightly into the bloodstream and acts topically on the lining of the colon to supress tissue inflammation before being eliminated in the stool.

You may be wondering why it is not possible simply to take 5-ASA without the sulfapyridine. The reason is that the 5-ASA molecule (without its sulfapyridine carrier molecule) is absorbed in the upper small intestine and is excreted in the urine before it can reach the colon and exert its beneficial effect. Recently, preparations of 5-ASA have been developed that reach the small intestine and colon in active form. These medications are the subject of the next section.

Side Effects of Sulfasalazine

Some side effects of sulfasalazine are distressing but not serious. These include headache, nausea, loss of appetite, and indigestion. The use of an enteric-coated tablet may prevent some of these digestive symptoms. These side effects can often be eliminated if therapy with sulfasalazine is begun at smaller than usual doses followed by gradually increased doses. For example, therapy can begin with a dose of 1 tablet twice daily for 2–3 days with a gradual increase to 4–6 or 8 tablets/day.

Side effects can often be eliminated if therapy with sulfasalazine is begun at smaller than usual doses followed by gradually increased doses.

Fever and rash are serious side effects that indicate an allergic reaction to sulfasalazine. It was once thought that these symptoms made it impossible to use sulfasalazine in further treatment. Experience has now shown that fever and/or rash can often be prevented if the medication is restarted in extremely small doses. This process is called **desensitization.** Initial doses can be as small as one quarter of a tablet (or 1cc of the oral suspension) daily for several days. The dose is then increased to one quarter of a tablet twice daily for several days and slowly to larger amounts. Complete blood counts and platelet counts are recommended at some periodic interval during this process. If fever or rash returns during this gradual process, further therapy with sulfasalazine should be stopped.

In addition, sulfasalazine may cause infertility in men who are using the medication for periods of time. However, this effect is temporary and fertility is restored when sulfasalazine is stopped. Other potentially serious side effects include acute pancreatitis (inflammation of the pancreas), hepatitis, and pneumonitis (inflammation of the lungs). If any of these side effects occur, sulfasalazine should be stopped. Fortunately, these adverse reactions are extremely rare.

Sulfasalazine does not usually have any adverse effects on pregnancy and can be continued safely throughout the pregnancy and into the nursing period. (Chapter 12 discusses the use of sulfasalazine and other IBD medications during pregnancy.)

A very serious side effect caused by sulfasalazine involves the bone marrow itself. Sulfasalazine may suppress the formation of all three types of blood cells found in the bone marrow: white blood cells, red blood cells, and platelets. Fortunately, bone marrow toxicity caused by sulfasalazine occurs very rarely. It can be discovered quickly with one simple blood test—the complete blood count (CBC). A CBC should be obtained at some regular interval during the first few months of

treatment and then at some periodic interval. If bone marrow depression is found, sulfasalazine should be stopped immediately, and should never be prescribed again. You should be careful to avoid *all* other medications containing sulfa.

Sulfasalazine may also cause damage to red blood cells after they have been manufactured by the bone marrow. In some people, red blood cells react to the presence of sulfa by undergoing a premature breakdown called **hemolysis.** If hemolysis occurs, sulfasalazine will usually be stopped.

The Aminosalicylates in IBD

As discussed above, 5-ASA, known by the generic name mesalamine, is the active component of sulfasalazine. Enema and suppository forms of 5-ASA are now available to treat ulcerative colitis limited to the rectum (proctitis) and the lower colon (proctosigmoiditis). These forms of 5-ASA come into direct contact with the inflamed bowel. This topical treatment with 5-ASA can prevent relapses of ulcerative colitis once the inflammation has subsided; it may also be helpful in Crohn's disease that is limited to the rectum and lower colon.

Oral forms of 5-ASA appear to be effective in treating active ulcerative colitis and in preventing relapses once the colitis is in remission. Initial studies of these agents in treating Crohn's disease suggest that 5-ASA is effective not only when Crohn's disease is active but may prevent relapses if used promptly after remission has been achieved.

Preparations and Doses
An enema preparation (Rowasa®), containing 4 grams of 5-ASA in a 60 ml container, is now available in the U.S. When using this enema, you are instructed to insert the exposed tip of the plastic container into the rectum and gently squeeze the container to allow fluid into the rectum. By trial and error, each person can

determine how firmly and rapidly to squeeze the container to permit the delivery of the fluid without stimulating the urge to evacuate. Your doctor will probably prescribe the enemas at bedtime in the hope that you can retain the fluid through the night. It may take several weeks of nightly use of the enema to calm the inflammation. Enemas can then be taken every second or third night to prevent recurrence of inflammation. Suppository forms of 5-ASA to treat inflammation limited to the rectum are also available. These are quite effective in relieving local inflammation.

A variety of oral forms of 5-ASA have been developed that can deliver the medication to the lower small intestine and colon. One preparation, olsalazine (Dipentum®), contains two 5-ASA molecules bonded together. Bacteria in the intestine break the bond and release the active medication. At the present time, Dipentum® is the only oral preparation of 5-ASA approved for use in the U.S. by the Food and Drug Administration (FDA). It has been approved to maintain a remission in ulcerative colitis for people who are unable to take sulfasalazine. The usual dose is 500 mg (2 capsules) twice a day with meals.

Other oral preparations awaiting FDA approval use either an acrylic-based resin or cellulose beads to coat 5-ASA. This ensures that the drug is not released until it reaches the less acid environments of the lower small intestine and colon. Although these forms of 5-ASA are available in Canada and in parts of Europe, they have not yet been approved for sale in the U.S.

Almost 90 percent of people with IBD who cannot take sulfasalazine because of intolerance or an allergic reaction can safely take 5-ASA.

Side Effects of 5-ASA

Almost 90 percent of people with IBD who cannot take sulfasalazine because of intolerance or an allergic reaction can safely take 5-ASA. However, about 10 percent of those allergic to sulfasalazine may have a similar reaction to 5-ASA, so this medication may have to be used carefully at first. Serious but rare side effects of both topical and oral forms of 5-ASA include pancreatitis, pericarditis (inflammation of the lining of the heart), pneumonitis, and a worsening of colitis. Rowasa® enemas may cause anal irritation that may be the result of sulfites in the fluid delivering 5-ASA. Dipentum® may cause a watery diarrhea that is unrelated to IBD.

Corticosteroids in IBD

Corticosteroids are effective in the treatment of both Crohn's disease and ulcerative colitis. These drugs reduce tissue inflammation and thereby relieve symptoms such as diarrhea, rectal bleeding, abdominal pain and fever. These drugs also relieve other "systemic" symptoms associated with IBD, including joint pains and inflammation of the skin and eyes. After ulcerative colitis has been brought under control, maintenance therapy with low-dose corticosteroids does not prevent a flare-up. (You will recall that maintenance therapy with sulfasalazine or 5-ASA can prevent a flare up in ulcerative colitis). In Crohn's disease, maintenance therapy with corticosteroids does not prevent a flare-up, nor does it prevent a recurrence of the disease after surgery.

At times in both ulcerative colitis and in Crohn's disease, corticosteroids and sulfasalazine or 5-ASA are administered simultaneously. However, it is not known whether these combinations are more beneficial than a corticosteroid agent administered by itself.

Preparations and Doses

Corticosteroids can be administered in many forms. Oral preparations include prednisone and methylprednisolone (Medrol®) tablets. The medication can also be given by intravenous or intramuscular injection in the form of hydrocortisone, prednisolone, or methylprednisolone (Solu-Medrol®), and through the rectum as an enema or foam. Intravenous or intramuscular steroids are used when patients are unable to take oral medication or are acutely ill and need to respond quickly to treatment. Corticosteroid enemas and foams are very helpful in healing active inflammation of the rectum and the lower colon.

A related medication sometimes used in IBD is corticotropin (ACTH). ACTH is a hormone secreted by the pituitary gland to stimulate the release of cortisol, the body's own form of corticosteroid, from the adrenal gland. ACTH is available only as an intramuscular or intravenous preparation and is as effective as corticosteroids in reducing inflammation. Some physicians feel that, in some situations, ACTH may be even more effective and may prevent the suppression of the adrenal gland sometimes caused by synthetic corticosteroids.

Corticosteroid enemas, foams, and suppositories are especially helpful in relieving uncomfortable rectal symptoms, particularly **tenesmus.** Tenesmus is triggered by rectal inflammation and is relieved only temporarily by passing a small amount of liquid stool. Steroid preparations inserted into the rectum reduce inflammation and promote healing in two ways. First, they come into direct contact with the inflamed bowel surface. Second, they are partially absorbed into the system, much like steroids taken by mouth. These preparations are helpful in ulcerative colitis and in Crohn's disease affecting the rectum and lower colon.

Corticosteroids available for rectal use include suppositories, rectal foam, and enemas. A suppository such as Anusol-HC,® which contains 10 mg of hydrocortisone, is easy to insert, and may be effective for mild proctitis. Rectal preparations that include corticosteroids as a foam include Cortifoam,® which contains 80 mg of hydrocortisone with each application, and Proctofoam-HC,® which contains 5 mg of hydrocortisone with each application. Foam preparations come with an applicator, making it easy to insert them into the rectum. Since these foams contain mostly air, they do not cause the urge to evacuate and can be easily retained.

When active inflammation extends well into the sigmoid colon, foams may not be dispersed deep enough to coat this tissue, and enemas may be needed. The most familiar of these products is Cortenema,® which contains 100 mg of hydrocortisone in a 60 ml container. These enemas can be used in an identical manner to the Rowasa® enemas. It is usually best to take these enemas at bedtime in the hope that you will retain them through the night. They can also be administered in the morning if symptoms are severe enough to require therapy twice daily. It is important to remember that people taking rectal steroids absorb a portion of this medication and may develop some of the same side effects as those who take steroids by mouth.

Side Effects of Corticosteroids

Serious side effects caused by corticosteroid therapy do not happen often but when they do, they are a cause for concern. Steroids can sometimes cause thinning of the bones (osteoporosis), high blood sugar, high blood pressure, cataracts, the increased likelihood of infections, and serious personality changes. Less serious side effects can still be troubling; these include loss of hair, acne, rounding of the face, fluid retention and stretch marks over the abdomen. The potential for most side effects diminishes as the dose of corticosteroids is reduced and usually disappears completely when the medication is discontinued. An exception is **aseptic necrosis** of the hip, a complication of the continuous use of high-dose steroids. This complication can appear long after steroids are discontinued and may require surgery and cause difficulty in walking.

The potential for most side effects diminishes as the dose of corticosteroids is reduced and usually disappears completely when the medication is discontinued.

Experience has shown that when corticosteroids are administered every other day, the potential for serious side effects is minimized. This method of treatment has been particularly helpful with children and adolescents who are often greatly troubled by the side effects of steroids. However, alternate-day therapy may not be possible if the disease process is very active.

Another possible side effect of corticosteroid therapy is insufficiency of the adrenal glands. Our adrenal glands normally manufacture small amounts of a natural corticosteroid hormone which helps the body to respond to any "stress," such as infection or surgery. When synthetic steroids are given as medication, the body's production of its own steroids temporarily shuts down. The goal of steroid therapy is gradually to decrease the dose so that the adrenal gland can begin working again. In some people, this may take some time and the adrenal gland may not function normally for six months to a year after steroids have been stopped. People with adrenal insufficiency may require an additional "boost" of corticosteroids if they develop infections or need surgery.

Immunosuppressive Agents in IBD

Immunosuppressives are substances that change the body's normal immune response to disease or to antigens (foreign substances within the body). They have been used to treat the so-called autoimmune diseases—diseases in which the tissues are attacked by the body's own antibodies—and to prevent the rejection of transplanted organs. Immunosuppressive agents such as azathioprine (Imuran®) and 6-mercaptopurine (6-MP or Purinethol®) have a limited role in the treatment of ulcerative colitis. This is because sulfasalazine, 5-ASA, and corticosteroids are usually quite effective and because physicians remain concerned about potential side effects of this group of medications (see below). For these reasons, immunosuppressive medications are not generally used alone in the treatments of ulcerative colitis. Some physicians prescribe these medications when ulcerative colitis requires large doses of corticosteroids for a long time to control the symptoms. In this case, the immunosuppressive drug may permit a gradual reduction in the dose of steroids and reduce the possibility of side effects caused by continuous high dose steroid therapy.

Immunosuppressive medications may take as long as three to six months to achieve results.

In Crohn's disease, either 6-MP or azathioprine is often administered together with sulfasalazine and/or corticosteroids. Using immunosuppressives in this way often improves symptoms and helps to close fistulas. In one study, fistulas closed completely in about 40 percent of patients and showed significant improvement in an additional 25 percent. After improvement of symptoms, the dose of corticosteroids can be reduced and at times discontinued completely while the immunosuppressive drug is continued. Immunosuppressive medications may take as long as three to six months to achieve results. For this reason, sulfalazine and/or corticosteroids are usually continued during this period. Once immunosuppressive therapy is stopped, relapses may occur but these often respond to reintroduction of the medication.

A different immunosuppressive drug, cyclosporin, has been used successfully in patients with organ transplants and shows promise as a treatment for both Crohn's disease and ulcerative colitis. The advantage of this medication is that it acts quickly, with good results usually seen within two weeks. However, because of the potential for serious toxicity, most physicians are awaiting results of further trials of this drug before using it extensively in treating IBD.

Preparations and Doses

Azathioprine is broken down by the liver to 6-MP, its active component. Most physicians believe that the two drugs are equally effective and can be used interchangeably. The usual starting dose for either medication is 50 mg (1 tablet/day). This dose may be raised to 1.5 mg/kg of body weight/day if there is no improvement at lower doses. If you are taking immunosuppresives, it is important to stay in very close contact with your physician to prevent the development of serious side effects (see below). Blood tests must be obtained at regular intervals, including a complete blood count (CBC) and platelet count. You must not assume that the physician receives a report of each blood test and that it is safe to continue this medication; it is your responsibility to receive a verbal communication either from the physician or from one of his staff that the results of tests permit you to continue with this medication.

Side Effects of Immunosuppressives

Immunosuppressive agents may cause a reduction in the number of certain blood cells, namely white blood cells and platelets formed in the bone marrow. An abnormally low number of white blood cells (cells that fight infection) may allow a serious infection to develop. A low platelet count may cause bleeding. Fortunately, a routine periodic CBC and platelet count can alert the physician that the medication should be reduced or stopped altogether. Other side effects that occur very rarely include nausea, fever, rash, pancreatitis and hepatitis. In addition, cyclosporin may cause damage to kidney function and result in hypertension. While there has been no evidence of increased development of cancer among patients with IBD who have received immunosuppressive agents for intervals of 15 to 20 years, people who remain on immunosuppressive therapy should keep in close touch with their doctors.

Antibiotics

Metronidazole

Metronidazole (Flagyl®) is an antibiotic used to treat a variety of parasitic and bacterial infections. It does not appear to be effective in active ulcerative colitis, although one small study suggests that it may prevent flare-ups of ulcerative colitis. In Crohn's disease, metronidazole has been successful in treating severe fissures and fistulas around the anus, as well as the general symptoms of Crohn's colitis. It does not appear to be as effective when Crohn's disease is limited to the small intestine. Metronidazole is probably beneficial because of its antibacterial activity, but there may be some immunologic properties of this medication as well.

Metronidazole is usually taken by mouth in doses of 10–20 mg/kg of body weight per day. Response to the drug may take several weeks. If symptoms return when metronidazole is reduced or discontinued, restarting the medication usually brings relief.

One important side effect occurring at high doses (and rarely at low doses) is numbness of the lower legs and feet. Most of the time, these symptoms disappear when the dose is lowered or the medication is stopped. In a few cases, however, these symptoms persist indefinitely. Other side effects include nausea, a metallic taste in the mouth, discoloration of the urine and loss of appetite. As with many medications, there is always a concern about possible long-term side effects, including the development of cancer. However, there is no evidence to date that metronidazole causes cancer in humans. No other serious long-term side effects of metronidazole have been identified.

Ciprofloxacin

When metronidazole is not effective or cannot be tolerated, ciprofloxacin (Cipro®) has been reported in one uncontrolled study as a useful alternative in treating severe perianal disease. As with metronidazole, symptoms often return when the medication is stopped.

Other Antibiotics

Antibiotics are best used to treat the infections that often complicate ulcerative colitis or Crohn's disease. Once the lining of the small or large intestine is damaged, bacteria may penetrate the bowel wall and cause either a local or systemic infection. When a flare-up of disease is associated with a high fever and other signs of infection, an antibiotic or combination of antibiotics is usually given intravenously. Because steroids may mask important signs of infection such as fever, antibiotics are often used during the first 7 to 10 days of treatment with corticosteroid agents.

Among several side effects that may occur with antibiotic therapy, one that is easily recognized is a secondary yeast infection of the mouth and throat called thrush. This infection is caused by an organism called *Candida albicans* and occurs more often in people who are quite ill and are receiving multiple medications, including antibiotics and/or steroids. Whitish plaques appear on the lining of the cheeks, tongue or throat. There may also be a sore throat or pain in the upper chest during swallowing. This usually means that the infection has spread to the esophagus. If you are receiving antibiotics and/or corticosteroids, make it a point to check for these signs. Treatment consists of oral solutions that can be gargled and swallowed several times a day.

Other Potential Agents

A variety of unrelated medications have shown promise in preliminary studies in treating IBD. Methotrexate, used for a number of years to treat various cancers, psoriasis, and some types of arthritis, appears to be effective in treating active ulcerative colitis and Crohn's disease and may prove to be useful in preventing relapses of these diseases. Chloroquine, an antimalarial drug, showed enough promise in treating a few patients with active ulcerative colitis to warrant an extended controlled trial using a related drug, hydroxychloroquine (Plaquenil®). The results of that trial are expected soon. Fish oils may reduce the production of a chemical partly responsible for the inflammatory reaction in colitis. One trial of fish oil in treating ulcerative colitis showed that it may be helpful in reducing symptoms. A more powerful medication with properties similar to fish oil is now being studied. Although the early studies of these agents are encouraging, more work needs to be done before they can be given routinely.

Antidiarrheal Agents

Diarrhea is a major symptom in IBD. It is important to reduce the number of loose bowel movements in order to promote better sleep, encourage food intake, and allow daily actities to continue normally. At the same time, overuse of medications to reduce diarrhea may lead to serious complications. As a general rule, you should try to aim for a modest reduction in the number of stools rather than total elimination of the problem.

As a general rule, you should try to aim for a modest reduction in the number of stools rather than total elimination of the problem.

There are several categories of drugs that can help to relieve diarrhea. In IBD, the substances used most often to control diarrhea are narcotics or synthetic narcotics. Examples of these are codeine, diphenoxylate (Lomotil®) and loperamide (Imodium®). Loperamide has an important second property of tightening the anal sphincter and helping to prevent incontinence. A second group of antidiarrheal drugs increases the intestinal absorption of fluid and electrolytes. Corticosteroids also have this property and improvement in diarrhea with these drugs is probably a reflection of this action as well as a reduction in tissue imflammation. Other medications that may help to improve absorption of fluid and electrolytes are clonidine and the phenothiazines. These medications also have significant side effects and should be used cautiously.

Cholestyramine (Questran®) is another medication that may help to reduce diarrhea when there is either extensive inflammation of the terminal ileum or surgical removal of a portion of the terminal ileum.

How a New IBD Drug Reaches the Market

A new prescription drug reaches the market through a long and arduous process which begins in the laboratory. Basic researchers in biochemistry and pharmacology develop substances which have *biological* activity—that is, they have an effect on living tissues. It then becomes the responsibility of the pharmaceutical company to insure that these compounds have *therapeutic* or beneficial activity in humans. This is accomplished through lengthy animal studies and through studies using actual patients, called controlled clinical trials.

Through these controlled trials, the effects of the new drug on IBD patients, for example, would be compared with the effects of a placebo on another group of IBD patients. (A placebo is a non-drug made to appear in every way like the test drug, but without its biological effects.) In this way, response to the new drug can be measured against the effect of simply giving treatment. Until the study is completed, the investigator is "blinded" and is unaware of which patients are receiving the actual drug. Of course, participants in clinical trials of any new drug are advised of the risks and benefits of the study and sign an informed consent signifying their willingness to participate.

When clinical testing is completed, a process that usually takes several years, the pharmaceutical company prepares a New Drug Application (NDA) for submission to the U.S. Food and Drug Administration (FDA). The NDA must contain all of the data accumulated during laboratory and clinical testing of the drug, including response to the drug, toxicity, and any adverse effects. If the data are accepted and the drug is approved, the company must still submit interval reports of any adverse effects that may come to light after approval.

Cholestyramine is a nonabsorbable resin that binds bile salts and other materials in the small intestine. When absorption of bile salts is incomplete (a result of disease or surgical removal of the terminal ileum), unabsorbed bile salts enter the colon and cause it to secrete an excessive amount of fluid and electrolytes (disolved mineral salts). Cholestyramine prevents this diarrhea by binding these bile salts before they reach the colon. One package or one scoop (4 grams) dissolved in a glass of water or fruit juice before breakfast is usually all that is needed to control diarrhea. (Apple juice is especially effective in disguising the unpleasant taste.) Additional doses can be taken before lunch and dinner if needed. If diarrhea does not improve and if there is weight loss, cholestyramine should be discontinued. Since cholestyramine may bind to chemicals other than bile acids, it should be taken one to two hours before or after other medications. Recently, cholestyramine became available in a flavored resin bar, under the name Cholebar.®

Occasionally, diarrhea alternates with constipation and a feeling of incomplete evacuation. In such cases, 1 tablespoon of a bulking agent containing psyllium (Metamucil,® Citrucel®) taken in juice or water in the morning or early evening may help the problem.

The most serious side effect of narcotics and other agents used to control diarrhea and cramps is the development of toxic megacolon. Toxic megacolon is a paralysis of the motor activity of the colon that causes distention (stretching of the bowel wall) and can lead to perforation. Early symptoms include an increase in abdominal pain, swelling and tenderness of the abdomen, and persistent fever. There are also fewer bowel movements, a situation that ordinarily would be interpreted as a sign of improvement. Toxic megacolon is a potentially very serious condition that requires hospitalization.

Narcotic Dependence in IBD

The use of narcotic substances to control pain and diarrhea creates several serious problems for the person with IBD. First, narcotic use reduces symptoms without treating the underlying illness. Second, these drugs cause the body to become tolerant and to require larger and larger doses to achieve the same result. Third, narcotic use often creates a separate set of bowel symptoms ("narcotic bowel syndrome") superimposed on IBD, which may become a separate problem, requiring treatment in the hospital.

We do not know how common narcotic dependence is in IBD. In a recent study of 43 IBD patients referred to a psychiatrist, 30 percent were found to be dependent on some form of addicting medication. While this high percentage is probably not typical of all people with IBD, the best estimate is that about one in 20 people will develop some problem with drug dependence in the course of their therapy.

The best way to combat this problem is to have some knowledge about how these drugs can be used safely and to work with a single physician who is also knowledgeable about this. Often, people with IBD have several doctors involved in their care: a family doctor, a gastroenterologist and, at times, a surgeon. The most important factor preventing narcotic dependence is to "appoint" one physician in the team to be the only one to prescribe narcotics. This allows good monitoring of the need for narcotics.

Often, the earliest signs of addiction are known only to the person taking the narcotic, and he or she will often deny them.

Narcotics commonly used for pain are codeine, meperidine (Demerol®) and oxycodone (Percocet® and Percodan®). For more severe pain and usually only in the hospital, injectable narcotics are used; these include pentazocaine (Talwin®), opium alkaloids, and morphine sulfate. These drugs can be used safely without causing drug dependence as long as they are carefully monitored by a physician, the dose gradually reduced, and the medication discontinued when the acute episode resolves. When pain lasts longer than two to three weeks, narcotics are not a good regular treatment because of the development of tolerance and the risk of drug dependence. In addition, the regular use of narcotics can actually *increase* a person's sensitivity to pain. Persistent pain may indicate a need to change the medications used to treat IBD.

For diarrhea, the situation is somewhat different. The drugs commonly used are diphenoxylate (Lomotil®), deodorized tincture of opium, and codeine. The risk of addiction is still present with these drugs, but it is less than with the other narcotics.

Recognizing the Signs of Drug Dependence

The signs of drug dependence should be familiar to all IBD patients and their families. Usually, the earliest sign is preoccupation with the drug (e.g. counting the time until the next dose) or use of the drug for reasons other than to control pain and diarrhea (for example as a sleeping medication). The next danger signs to watch for are the use of increasing doses or a shortening of the time interval between doses. At this point, withdrawal symptoms (anxiety, cramps, sweating, irritability) may be felt if a dose is missed. These symptoms indicate a physical addiction. If this situation is allowed to progress, the person may seek to obtain more medication (commonly by "losing" prescriptions or consulting other doctors with the intention of obtaining a narcotic). Family members or friends may begin to notice that the person is doing less, "looks spacey," and may have slurred speech. These signs should be discussed with the doctor immediately. Often, the earliest signs of addiction are known only to the person taking the narcotic, and he or she will often deny them. This is unfortunate because if detected early, drug dependence is not yet fully developed and can be more easily treated.

A word should be said about the use of narcotics by people with IBD who have had a prior drug problem or are still involved with drugs. Such a problem could be the use of cocaine, tranquilizers, alcohol, or even marijuana. At least one in 14 young people have such a problem and some of them develop IBD. It is crucial to let your physician know about this, even if drugs have not been a problem for years. If your doctor knows about this situation, he or she can use extra caution in prescribing narcotics.

Adjusting to an Ostomy

6

The purpose of this chapter is to help you adjust to living with a conventional ileostomy. Physical care and management of an ostomy is extremely important. You will have to learn a new method of having bowel movements which is not normal and yet allows you to be in control of your elimination. Even though you may have learned to live with chronic inflammatory bowel disease and have reached an understanding that surgery is necessary, actually having ostomy surgery may be a very emotional time. The fear of the unknown and lack of control all of us experience while in hospitals only adds to the reactions you may have when faced with ostomy surgery.

The myths and misconceptions about ostomies would fill volumes.

The decision to undergo surgery is a joint decision made by your gastroenterologist and surgeon and by you. The need for and timing of surgery depends on many factors: the severity of your disease, the presence of complications, your response to medical treatment, the side effects of your medications, and the extent to which the disease is interrupting your daily life. In some instances, surgery will have to be performed as an emergency; more often it is performed electively because medications have failed to control your symptoms. If this is the case, you must play a major role in the decision-making about your surgery. You should discuss all aspects of the surgery, including the reasons for operation, the possible complications, and the anticipated outcome with your surgeon so that you will feel satisfied with the decision. If you are not

convinced that all possible medical means have been tried, you may want to seek an opinion from another gastroenterologist. Most people are more accepting of surgery, especially an ileostomy, if they have discussed and considered all the alternatives.

In many cases, an ostomy will not be needed. In some instances, an ostomy may be required only temporarily. For those with ulcerative colitis, surgical techniques have been developed that avoid the use of ostomy equipment altogether. These include the continent ileostomy (Kock pouch) and the ileoanal anastomosis ("pull-through operation"). (These operations are discussed at length in the book *Treating IBD* and in other publications available from the CCFA, listed in the Appendix. A chapter on coping with a pull-through operation follows this one.) In Crohn's disease, usually only the diseased portion of bowel is removed. Because the rectum is usually spared, the two ends of the bowel can often be joined together, making an ileostomy unnecessary.

If a permanent ileostomy *is* necessary, the decision to have surgery can be a difficult one. Many stories abound about ostomy surgery and living with an ostomy; the myths and misconceptions about ostomies would fill volumes. In the past, having ostomy surgery was not considered a positive option, largely because of the scarcity of good ostomy equipment and health professionals to care for people after ostomy surgery. Today, there are modern ostomy appliances, enterostomal therapists (E.T.s), and support groups available to help people adjust to life with an ostomy. In addition, people seem more able to discuss bowel function today than in the past. Thus, many of the concerns previously held by ostomates no longer apply.

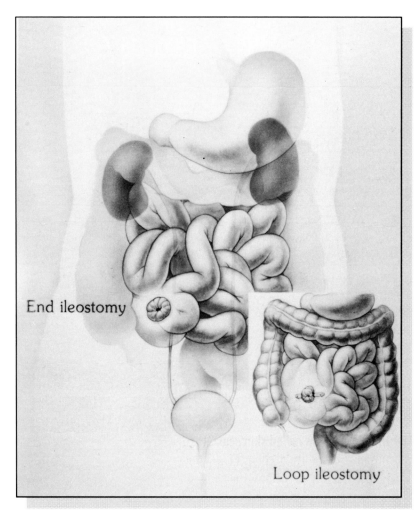

End ileostomy

Loop ileostomy

An ileostomy.
Courtesy of R. McLeod, IBD Unit, Mt. Sinai Hospital, Toronto.

It is natural that you will have concerns about ostomy surgery since you are facing not only an operative procedure but also a major change in your body image. Many people are afraid to have surgery if it means having an ileostomy and may delay surgery for prolonged periods of time. After surgery these same people are usually extremely happy that they have had the operation and regret not having had it sooner. They feel that having an ostomy is a small price to pay for improved physical health and well-being, not to mention the freedom from taking medications such as steroids. The ostomy may be an inconvenience but rarely does it interfere with normal activities.

Before you can learn how to care for your ostomy, it is important to understand the new words you will be using to describe your ostomy and the items you will use in its care.

Some Ostomy Terms and What They Mean

Stoma—This is the visible portion of the intestine that protrudes through an opening on the skin. A stoma is formed by bringing the end of the small bowel or large bowel through the abdominal wall and turning it back on itself like a cuff. It is normal for the stoma to be a bright red color; it is moist to the touch because the inner intestinal lining normally produces a mucous substance. There are no sensory nerve endings in the stoma, even though its bright red color may make you think it might be painful. However, the motor nerves in the stoma are still connected to the bowel, and the slight motion you will sometimes see in the stoma is the usual motion of the bowel **(peristalsis)** as it propels contents through the intestinal tract.

Ileostomy—An ileostomy is an opening into the ileum or lower part of the small intestine. The drainage from the stoma is called feces, stool or **effluent.** Ileostomy effluent contains digestive enzymes that are normally present in the small bowel to help break down food products. Because these enzymes are extremely irritating, the skin must be protected with an appliance. The ileostomy discharges effluent at unpredictable times but most frequently after eating. Most people report that they need to empty the pouch four to six times a day, generally after meals and before going to bed. The effluent will be very liquid immediately after surgery but it will thicken as your diet becomes more varied.

Colostomy—A colostomy is an opening into the large bowel that is usually brought out through the skin on the lower left side of the abdomen. It may be either temporary or permanent. A colostomy is permanent if the lower portion of the bowel and rectum are removed. The stool from a colostomy tends to be more formed than that from an ileostomy and the digestive enzymes usually have been absorbed or deactivated by the time the stool passes through the ascending colon. You may hear of people with colostomies irrigating or giving themselves an enema through the colostomy stoma to control their bowel movements. Generally, colostomy irrigation is *not* recommended for people with Crohn's colitis because the disease process can recur and the bowel may be irritated by the irrigation.

Pouches (appliances, bags)— These are external collecting devices used following ostomy surgery. Pouches are odor proof; this means that they will contain the normal odor of the stool until the bottom is opened for emptying. Appliances are available in a variety of sizes and styles. You can choose one that will fit your stoma and your body contours and will not be visible under your clothing.

Some people like to flush the pouch with water once a day, although this is not required. It is important to clean the spout with toilet tissue after each emptying. A small clamp is used to close the bottom of the pouch; the edge of the pouch folds up into the clamp leaving an exposed edge. If stool is left on this edge or if the clamp is dirty, there may be some odor. If gas is a problem, several appliances are available with charcoal filters. These filters deodorize the gas as it is released.

Skin Barriers—Products which provide a solid barrier to protect the skin around the stoma. The most commonly used skin barrier is a pectin-based wafer. These wafers are used to protect the skin from breakdown and to promote healing when minor irritations occur. The wafer should have an opening cut into it for the stoma. Many of the solid wafers are also available in paste forms and can be used to fill in small creases or cover any exposed skin when the opening is a little too large. Many appliances are available with pectin-based wafers already attached.

Liquid skin barriers called skin sealants are also available and are used to protect the skin under tape. It is extremely important to keep the skin in excellent condition under and around the pouch to prevent irritation.

Ostomate—This is a general term used to refer to people who have undergone ostomy surgery. Many doctors and nurses will use it to refer collectively to people who have had ostomy surgery. However, it is important to remember that you were (and are) a person before you were an ostomate!

Some Common Concerns about Ostomies

Odor is a major concern of most people, especially before they have the surgery. Surveys of ileostomates suggest that between 30 and 40 percent of ostomates have problems with odor. In most instances, however, these are minor problems and can be controlled and managed with proper

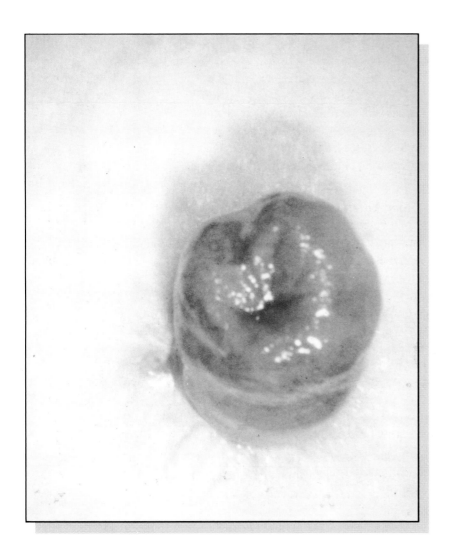

The stoma after surgery.

appliances and some dietary modifications. The pouches which are available today are odor-proof and odor-resistant. Products are available which can be inserted into the appliance to neutralize odor. Charcoal filter systems are also available to allow control of odor associated with the release of gas from the pouch. Some people choose to take bismuth subgallate by mouth to control odor. As with anything taken by mouth, you should consult with your enterostomal therapy nurse or doctor before taking it.

Odor can also be controlled by watching your diet. In particular, you should avoid certain foods that produce gas, such as vegetables in the cabbage family, asparagus, onions, melons, dried beans and peas, spicy foods, beer, cheese and milk products. If you enjoy these foods and do not wish to eliminate them from your diet, you can eat them in moderation or when you are planning to be at home. Yogurt, buttermilk and fresh parsley may actually decrease odor in the pouch.

Odor can also be a sign of a leaking pouch seal. If you are wearing an odor-proof system and you suddenly notice an odor, check your pouch seal to make sure it is intact. You should also double check your clamp and the edge of the pouch.

Skin care is extremely important for the ostomate. The skin around the stoma (peristomal skin) should be healthy and free of irritation. Cleaniness is important and will usually prevent most problems. The pouch should be changed every four to six days or more frequently during warm weather. It is important that you change your pouch routinely before it leaks. If there is any hair around the stoma, it should be clipped since shaving irritates the skin surface. When removing the appliance, take care not to pull out skin hairs.

Despite excellent care of the stoma and peristomal skin, you may experience occasional skin irritations. Most commonly, these are yeast infections or sensitivity reactions to the appliance barrier or tape. If this happens, an enterostomal therapy nurse can be extremely helpful in suggesting measures to eradicate the problem. It is important to keep wearing the appliance since irritation will worsen if there is leakage of stool onto the skin.

Diet is an area that concerns every person with a new ostomy. For six to eight weeks following surgery, you may be kept on a low residue diet that eliminates bulky and hard-to-digest foods. Gradually, you can begin to add new foods until you have resumed your normal healthy diet. If some foods still bother you, you can eliminate them from your meals or eat them only in moderation.

Most ostomates experience only minor dietary restrictions. Some foods that cause occasional problems are coarse whole grain breads, nuts or seeds, seafood (lobster, shrimp and crab), some legumes (lentils, dried beans and dried peas) and fresh fruit with skins and membranes. Raw vegetables such as bamboo shoots, bean sprouts, sauerkraut, corn, okra, turnips, mushrooms and anything prepared with nuts or seeds also may be difficult to digest.

It is important that you chew your food well, eat slowly and avoid the use of straws. Chewing food well and eating slowly helps you digest your foods, especially bulky and hard-to-digest foods. Drinking through a straw increases the amount of air swallowed resulting in more intestinal gas.

Fluid intake is very important when you have an ileostomy. The colon is usually responsible for the absorption of water and salt from the stool. While the small intestine will increase its absorption of fluid and salt when the colon is removed, you will still need to make sure you take in enough fluids and salt to prevent dehydration. This is especially true during the summer months or when you exercise heavily. If you have the flu with diarrhea and vomiting, you may lose more fluids and electrolytes (mineral salts) than if you still had your colon in place. Gatorade® and other high electrolyte drinks may be very helpful as supplements to keep you from having symptoms of dehydration.

If part of your small intestine has been removed along with your colon (as in Crohn's disease), you may have further fluid and salt loss which could cause problems. In this situation, you may need to follow some dietary restrictions or take medication to slow down your bowel. Symptoms of dehydration include a feeling of weakness or light-headedness when you stand up, a tingling feeling in the fingers and toes, and a low output of urine.

Concerns about the Quality of Life

Many people with ostomies worry that they might not be able to wear clothes they are

---

Keeping Your Ostomy Clean

Taking a shower in the morning before you eat or drink anything is a good idea, since you can shower with the pouch on or off. It does not hurt the stoma to get shampoo and/or soap on it. For many people with ostomies, it feels good to rinse their skin without any adhesives on it. If you prefer to bathe in a tub, you should probably keep the pouch on in case the stoma becomes active. Special creams or soaps are not required to clean around the stoma; ordinary soap and water may be used as long as the soap is rinsed off well. Some people use wash cloths to clean around their stomas, while others use the thicker type of paper towels. Kleenex and toilet paper are too thin and will fall apart easily.

Diarrhea: A Problem for the Ostomate

Diarrhea can become a serious problem for the ileostomate. Dehydration and electrolyte imbalance can occur rapidly, often the result of superimposed infections, certain medications, a blockage, or emotional distress. Certain foods such as fried foods, spiced foods, beans, and raw fruits may cause watery stools for some people. Determining whether diarrhea is present may not be easy because the output from the ileostomy is already of a liquid consistency. If there is a noticeable increase in the amount of liquid output and the pouch needs to be emptied more frequently, this should be considered as probable evidence of diarrhea. In addition, diarrhea causes a decrease in urinary frequency because body fluids are being lost through the ileostomy. **The absence of any urine output indicates serious dehydration and warrants contacting your doctor immediately.**

The first treatment for diarrhea is to eliminate any food that may be causing the problem. As soon as the diarrhea begins, try to drink enough to replace one to one and one-half times the estimated ileostomy liquid output. Suggested replacements are an alternation between sweet tea and clear salty broth. Return to a low residue diet. Foods such as strained bananas, peanut butter and boiled rice will help to reduce the flow. Your physician may prescribe medication to help "turn off" the diarrhea.

accustomed to wearing. However, the ostomy appliance does not show under most clothing with the exception of bikinis and tight fitting clothes. Before surgery, the enterostomal therapy nurse will mark a suitable place on your abdomen where the surgeon will construct your stoma. The stoma is usually placed in a location where it does not interfere with clothing. This means that it is usually placed *below* the belt line so it cannot be irritated by belts or waist bands. If it is placed above the belt line, concealing the appliance may be difficult. Unfortunately, in some situations, this location cannot be avoided.

Your surgeon will encourage you to return to your normal routine including work, leisure activities, sports and hobbies once you have recovered from the operation. Recovery usually takes from four to six weeks. Resuming normal activities helps to increase your feelings of psychological well-being and mastery over the routines of your new ostomy. Only about 10 percent of ileostomates report any restrictions in participating sports, hobbies, and leisure activities. Some people with ostomies avoid swimming or sports which cause them to perspire a great deal and make it difficult to keep the appliance intact. To overcome this problem and to prevent leakage of stool, you can plan to change the appliance immediately following the activity.

Travelling with your new ostomy should not be difficult, provided you take precautions and so some advance planning. When you empty your appliance, you may require a sink; if so, try to choose a toilet facility where there is a sink and toilet within the same area away from public view. Overall, you may find that you have fewer problems travelling than you did before surgery. You can now empty your appliance at your convenience instead of worrying that you won't be able to reach a bathroom in time. For many ostomates, this freedom from anxiety is, by far, the greatest benefit of ostomy surgery.

Feelings about the Ostomy

Adapting to and living with an ostomy means learning to manage the physical changes and recognizing the emotional reactions you may have. It is normal to experience a time of emotional upheaval. First, there is the real, physical loss of a part of your body that cannot be seen; there is also the physical change in your elimination, the addition of the stoma on your abdomen, and in many cases, the closure of your rectum. There is no correct or right way to express your feelings about these changes. Some people go through stages of denial that anything is different, or anger that a cure or alternative operation is not available. Some people become depressed and have trouble eating, sleeping, and adapting to the changes.

Accepting these changes does not necessarily mean that you like having an ostomy, but it does mean that you can learn to live with the ostomy.

Accepting these many changes does not necessarily mean that you *like* having an ostomy, but it does mean that you can learn to live with the ostomy. You are still the same person you were before surgery. At first you will be very conscious of the pouch. You will notice every time stool begins to collect and you may find yourself emptying the pouch more often than necessary. This is a normal response to the newness of the pouch, the feel of the stool in the pouch, and fears about odor and leakage. As you become more active and more involved in other activities, you will become more accustomed to the pouch. You will learn when the pouch needs to be emptied based on its weight and feel. Soon you will be able to detect small signs that indicate it is time to change the system.

Intimate Relationships and Your Ostomy

You may be very concerned about how your spouse or lover will accept you now that you have a stoma. The pouch which is present on your abdomen can be hidden by clothes, but during intimate contact with your partner the pouch is evident and cannot always be hidden. The most important phase of intimacy is communication. Most people report that when they discuss the pouch, the stoma and the changes in their body image, they find a loving, accepting partner. Partners may be afraid they will hurt you if they give you a hug or put pressure on the stoma or pouch. You will need to teach them that normal pressure against the stoma is not painful or dangerous. Don't delay in discussing your feelings openly. Often your loved ones are feeling the same kind of emotions you are. These emotions should be shared.

Once you are feeling better, sexual relations can be resumed. Many find relations with their partner more pleasurable because of the lack of incapacitating disease. It is recommended that you start slowly, often with talking and close contact. During intercourse, you may want to experiment with different positions to find the one most comfortable for you. In addition, you should probably empty your pouch prior to sexual relations to minimize the risk of leakage.

Many patients are concerned about whether they may have children in the future. The answer is yes. During surgical removal of the rectum, there is a very minimal risk of damage to the nerves to the sexual organs in males which may lead to impotence or retrograde ejaculation. The chance that this might happen is less than 1 percent. Women with ostomies have no problem conceiving and, in most cases, the baby can be delivered vaginally.

An Ostomy Miscellany

- Skipping meals or limiting fluids does not cause a thickening of the discharge in the ostomy pouch or allow you to empty the pouch less often. This is dangerous and can cause dehydration.
- Foods that may lessen gas are applesauce, marshmallows and yogurt.
- To muffle the noise caused by gas escaping into the pouch, try placing your hand over the stoma and bending forward a little.
- Eating red foods like beets, red jello, tomato juice, or red-colored soda will cause the drainage in your ostomy pouch to turn red! (Don't worry, you're not bleeding.)
- Ileostomates are particularly susceptible to "blockages." Be alert for the signs of a blockage: pain, nausea and vomiting, decreased or increased ostomy output, and fever.
- To thicken the ileostomy output, some patients eat all the solid food at their meal first and *then* drink the fluids.
- Laxatives should *never* be taken by anyone with an ileostomy.
- If a belt causes problems around your stoma, wear suspenders!
- Tight jeans and other form fitting clothing, while doing wonders for your self-image, may rub against your stoma, causing it to bleed.
- When flying, it's a good idea to take the ileostomy supplies in a carry-on bag, since checked baggage may be lost or misplaced.

Talking about Your Ostomy

You will probably need someone to talk with about all the changes you are experiencing. Your enterostomal therapist can provide many opportunities for you to ask questions and to share your feelings. She will play a crucial role during your hospitalization, usually visiting you just before surgery to answer your questions and alleviate many of your anxieties. After surgery, she will visit you regularly, help you care for the appliance, and teach you how to care for it yourself when you leave the hospital. If necessary, arrangements can be made for home visits. In addition to the enterostomal therapist, your surgeon and gastroenterologist can provide information and support and can answer questions that you may have both before and after surgery.

You may also wish to meet someone who has had ostomy surgery and has learned to live successfully with the change. The United Ostomy Association (UOA) provides trained ostomy visitors who are available to come and talk with you before and after surgery. Your enterostomal therapy nurse or your physician can make the arrangements to have the visitor meet with you. The UOA also organizes self-help groups where people meet to discuss facts about ostomies and encourage each other to share the experience of living with an ostomy.

Your surgeon can also supply names and telephone numbers of patients who have undergone similar operations and have stomas. These patients are almost always quite willing to talk with you, knowing that you are experiencing what they experienced some time ago. There is nothing quite as encouraging as meeting and talking with someone like yourself who is healthy, active, and living life fully with an ostomy.

Coping with a
Pull-through Operation

7

People who have an operation for chronic ulcerative colitis almost always enjoy improved health and well-being as well as the freedom from taking regular medications. The classic operation for ulcerative colitis—total proctocolectomy with permanent ileostomy—cures the disease and is the standard against which all other operations are measured. However, the need for a permanent ileostomy and having to wear an ostomy appliance have discouraged some patients with ulcerative colitis; for this reason, continence-preserving procedures have been developed as alternatives to the traditional ileostomy. The most commonly performed of these operations is the **ileoanal anastomosis** with reservoir (pouch) or **"pull through"** operation, in which an intestinal pouch is fashioned from the patient's own ileum, and which allows for elimination of stool through the anal canal. (This operation is usually *not* performed on people with Crohn's disease because of the likelihood that the disease will recur in the pouch.)

No operation for ulcerative colitis is "perfect" since no procedure can restore a patient to a "normal" bowel pattern after years of debilitating disease. Patients with permanent ileostomies encounter a variety of stoma-related problems; fortunately most of these can be managed easily with the help of a skilled enterostomal therapist. Occasionally the stoma develops a problem such as a prolapse or hernia, which requires a separate surgical repair (See Chapter 6 for a discussion about the care of an ileostomy).

The ileoanal pull-through operations have a number of problems of their own. The pull-through operation is often done in two or three stages and each stage may be associated with major or minor complications. In the first one or two stages, the colon is removed, the diseased mucosa (inner lining) of the rectum is stripped from the underlying muscle, and a pouch or reservoir is constructed from the ileum and attached to the rectal muscle. A temporary ileostomy diverts feces away from the reservoir and allows the sutures (stitches) time to heal. Patients evacuate stool through the ileostomy into an appliance for several weeks to months. During this time, most people experience some discharge through the anus, consisting of mucus produced by the bowel and initially mixed with old blood or stool left over from before the operation. A small amount of bright red blood may also be seen, especially in the first week or two after the operation. This blood comes from the sutures or staple lines and usually stops by itself. If bleeding persists, or if more than 1 to 2 ounces are seen, it is advisable to contact your physician. Continued discharge of a small amount of mucus or stool is to be expected and is no cause for alarm. Unexpected drainage can be minimized by sitting on the toilet and releasing the fluid at a convenient time. Irritation of the skin around the anus can be avoided by wearing an absorbent pad in the underclothing. A protective barrier cream also may be applied to the skin (See page 59).

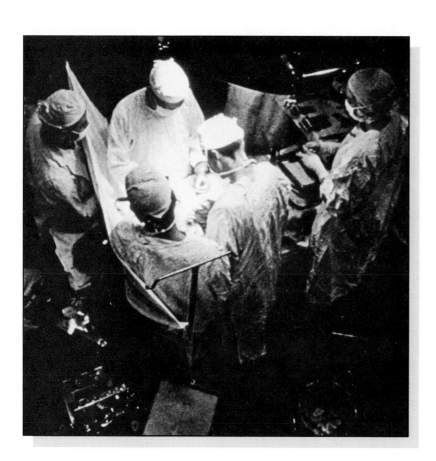

The Loop Ileostomy
After Surgery

The type of ileostomy constructed after the pull-through operation is called a **loop ileostomy.** This type of stoma or opening is formed in the part of the small intestine above the pouch. It is made by opening the bowel and turning back the functional part to form a stoma. The nonfunctional part of the small intestine leads to the new rectal pouch. The loop ileostomy stoma acts just like the ordinary end ileostomy stoma and may develop any of the usual stoma problems.

The stoma at the loop ileostomy looks somewhat like a peeled cherry tomato. It can be swollen at first, but within two to three weeks it will shrink in size to about the size of a button or a quarter. The stoma will always stay red in color like the inside of your mouth. It bleeds very easily just as gums bleed when teeth are brushed too vigorously. There may also be a supportive piece of plastic (a thin tube or a 1/4" flat piece of plastic) under the stoma to support it while the suture line under it heals. This supportive bridge is usually left in place from one to three weeks.

Before leaving the hospital, your enterostomal therapist will instruct you in the daily care of the ileostomy. You will learn how to empty and change the appliance (also called a pouch) and how to take care of the skin around the stoma. The pouch is usually changed twice a week. You will empty the pouch about four to six times each day, depending on your diet and fluid intake. There is a large variety of pouching systems on the market to fit the specific needs of each patient. There is no one best pouching system. The E.T. nurse will demonstrate which pouching system or systems best fits your needs.

When you are ready to go home, most hospitals will make a referral for an E.T.

It does not require great technical skill to care for an ileostomy. Most people find that the major hurdle is the psychological adjustment to the "new" way of going to the bathroom.

nurse or visiting nurse to continue teaching or provide support at home as you continue to adjust to the ostomy. It does not require great technical skill to care for an ileostomy. Most people find that the major hurdle is the psychological adjustment to the "new" way of going to the bathroom. Just about the time you have begun to feel comfortable with the ileostomy, it may be time to close the ileostomy and reconnect the bowel!

A Diet for Your Temporary Ileostomy

During the period of the temporary ileostomy, the diet should be slightly modified to avoid especially fibrous foods, such as string beans, Chinese vegetables, salads, corn, nuts, popcorn, etc. Small amounts of these foods are acceptable and should be chewed well. Too much undigestible bulk often causes a blockage of the bowel passage. Symptoms of a blockage include cramping which can progress to abdominal distension, vomiting and severe abdominal pain. The stoma output will decrease considerably, change to a clear yellow fluid, or may even increase. Partial blockage is common and usually temporary, resolving on its own after one or two hours. If there is no vomiting, you should sip small amounts of clear, non-carbonated fluids so you will not become dehydrated. If a blockage persists and progresses to full-blown obstruction with vomiting and pain, contact your physician immediately since this may require hospitalization.

Even if mild blockage occurs frequently, it is important to tell your doctor.

Caring for the Skin around the Anus

Another area of concern following the first stage of the pull-through operation is the care of the perianal skin (skin around the anus). Proper care of this area is extremely important because the mucus discharge can cause skin irritation.

The perianal skin must be cleaned and dried thoroughly after each mucus discharge. Using soft tissues or cotton balls and moistening these before wiping lessens friction on the skin. Hospital tissue or gauze is too abrasive on the perianal skin and colored or perfumed toilet paper can cause further irritation. Soaps are *not* recommended because they can be irritating and leave a residue that causes itching. The perianal skin needs to be rinsed thoroughly with water. Some people choose to use a plastic spray bottle, a hand-held shower spray or a douche set. To dry the skin, use a soft cloth, a "fan" made from a piece of cardboard, or simply a hand-held hair dryer on a low setting.

Moisture barrier ointments or creams applied to the perianal area can provide additional protection after the perianal skin has been dried. Products such as Desitin,® Triple Care Cream,® and Vaseline Constant Care® contain zinc oxide; those that are petrolatum-based (and are greasier) include Vaseline,® Peri-Care,® and Special Care Ointment.®

If you are away from home, such products as Tucks,® Baby Wipes,® or Wet Ones® are ideal for perianal cleansing. Drying is accomplished with gentle patting using plain white toilet paper. It is a good idea to carry a small tube of a moisture barrier ointment with you to apply after each cleansing.

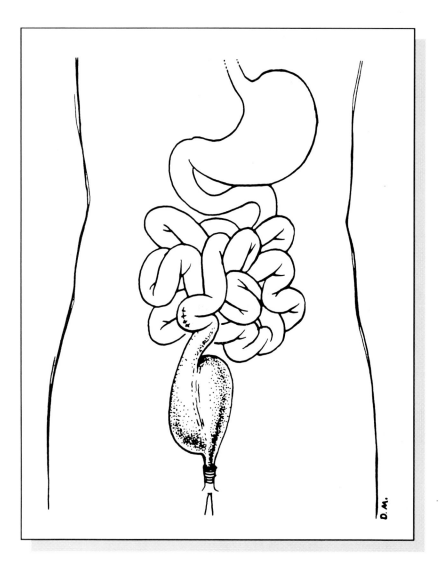

The intestine after a "pull-through" operation.
Courtesy of R. McLeod, IBD Unit, Mt. Sinai Hospital, Toronto.

Closure of the Ileostomy: What Happens Next?

The loop ileostomy is in place for several months, during which time the pouch heals and the anal muscle regains its tone. Once the loop ileostomy is closed, the stool will come through the normal pathway. At first there may be excessive diarrhea and moderate leakage between bowel movements, especially at night. Perianal skin care during this period is a must! With time, dietary manipulations, and the use of some medications, the bowel movements become more formed. This may be a slow process, taking a few weeks to several months or longer. The simplest treatments for this purpose are the bulking agents, such as Metamucil® or Konsyl,® Antidiarrheal medications such as Imodium,® Lomotil,® or codeine may also be needed to reduce stool frequency. You will have to experiment with the use of bulk-forming agents and antidiarrheal medications. Because each person is different, there is no "normal" or "average" bowel pattern after closure. After 6 to 12 months, most patients have an acceptable number of movements (usually 5 to 6) with better control, no bleeding, and considerably less urgency than before surgery.

Because each person is different, there is no "normal" or "average" bowel pattern after closure.

People who have persistent urgency, leakage, or worsening diarrhea may have developed "pouchitis." This condition may also occur long after the temporary stoma has been closed. The cause of pouchitis is uncertain, but many physicians think it is probably caused by an overgrowth of bacteria in the ileal reservoir, since it responds to treatment with antibiotics such as metronidazole, Cipro,® Augmentin,® or others. Enemas, preparations containing medications, such as Rowasa® or Cortenema,® may also be helpful in quieting the inflammation. Unfortunately, many people do not realize they have developed pouchitis and think that the urgency and diarrhea are to be expected after the operation. Fortunately, pouchitis can be recognized easily with a simple endoscopy procedure and usually responds quickly to appropriate medications. However, pouchitis may occasionally require prolonged and vigorous treatment.

Remember to discuss any unusual developments with your surgeon or gastroenterologist and don't be afraid to take medications to improve the functional result of your pull-through operation. The need for medication does not mean that the procedure has failed or that you are somehow inadequate. Many patients take medications soon after the operation and discontinue them later as the functional "new pathway" continues to improve.

Caring for the Perianal Skin after Closure

Because of the frequency of bowel movements after closure of the ileostomy, the perianal skin is especially vulnerable to additional breakdown. The liquid stool contains enzymes, substances secreted by the digestive tract to aid in the breakdown of food. Since these enzymes are irritating to the skin, you will need to use the same perianal care techniques after each bowel movement that you used before closure, with some modifications. In addition to plain water, Carrington Perineal Cleansing Foam® and Balneol® are good cleansing agents. As before, soaps should be avoided and the use of moisture barriers is recommended. It's a

good idea to wear white cotton underwear, since cotton absorbs perspiration and allows air to reach the skin. Minipads may be used during periods of incontinence to avoid soiling the underwear. If a pad is worn, it should be changed frequently to keep the skin dry.

What to Do about Perianal Irritation

Moderate irritation causes redness, burning, and itching around the perianal area; using the same cleansing and drying techniques used before closure of the ostomy should provide relief. Treatment may also include the application of an antibacterial/antifungal cream such as Aseptin® or Microguard.® A light sprinkling of pure cornstarch over the cream will also help to absorb the moisture.

If there is severe irritation, the skin around the anus will be red, raw, blistered and will weep fluid. You will experience severe burning and pain. To relieve these symptoms, try taking sitz baths in plain warm water and applying denatured calamine lotion two to three times per day to help dry the weepy skin. (To denature calamine lotion, let the bottle sit until the water comes to the top, then pour the water off. The lotion will be thicker and will dry faster.) Once the skin is healed, return to the treatment for moderate irritation. Occasionally, a few people experience perianal irritation that is extremely severe. They may need to use stronger antifungal preparations such as Mycostatin® powder, Mycolog® cream, or even corticosteroid products. These products require a prescription from a physician.

Most of the time perianal irritation clears up successfully with appropriate treatment. Remember that as bowel movements and leakage decrease, so does the problem of perianal irritation.

In summary, despite some problems during the first weeks and months after surgery, the ileoanal pull-through operation restores good health and controllable bowel movements. Medications like steroids are no longer necessary. Preoccupation with ill-health can now be replaced by attention to family, work, and the benefits of a full and active life.

What You Always Wanted to Know about IBD but Were Afraid to Ask

8

Most of the questions addressed in this chapter are dealt with in more detail in other sections of this book. Some issues, however, crop up so often and arouse so much concern that we thought it would be useful to bring them together and talk about them briefly all in one place.

1. *"How did I get this disease?"* Of all the questions people ask about IBD, most common is how they or their loved ones came to contract the disease. How? Why? Was it something I ate? Was it something I did or didn't do?

If these are the questions most frequently asked, they are also the toughest to answer. Nobody knows the cause or causes of ulcerative colitis or Crohn's disease. But there is one thing we know for sure. They are *not* caused by "nerves," they are *not* "psychosomatic," and there's *no such thing* as the "typical Crohn's or colitis personality." These pernicious myths have probably created more suffering from guilt than from all the pain, cramps, and diarrhea of IBD put together.

Why do so many people persist in thinking of ulcerative colitis and Crohn's disease as nervous diseases? It is probably because of the incorrect use of the term "colitis." For decades, doctors and lay people alike used to refer loosely and incorrectly to the stress-related condition, irritable bowel syndrome (IBS) as "colitis" ("spastic colitis," or "mucous colitis"). This erroneous terminology still creates needless confusion today. The irritable

bowel syndrome is a **functional** disorder that stems from a hyper-reactive muscular component of the bowel. There is some evidence that this condition may be inherited. Troublesome as it is, IBS is not a *true* "colitis" and it never causes any structural damage to the bowel wall. Ulcerative colitis and Crohn's disease, by contrast, are organic diseases that result in chronic injury to the intestinal tissues, including bleeding, ulceration, scarring, fistulas, and abscesses.

The immune systems of people with IBD seem to be predisposed to overract to the materials that the bowel ordinarily processes every day.

While the causes of ulcerative colitis and Crohn's disease are still unknown, an accumulating body of evidence seems to implicate some inherent defect in the control mechanisms that regulate the immune defense systems of the intestinal tract. In normal individuals, these immune systems are programmed to be tolerant of the masses of foreign proteins contained in the food and in the bacteria that swarm through our intestines. The immune systems of people with IBD, on the other hand, seem to be predisposed—perhaps in part genetically—to overract to the materials that the bowel ordinarily processes every day. In IBD, these immunologic alarms are set on hair-trigger, and they tend to provoke injurious inflammatory responses to dietary or bacterial stimuli that most people would find harmless. Treatments are therefore centered around medications like aminosalicylates (sulfasalazine and 5-ASA products), corticosteroids (prednisone), and immunosuppressives (6-MP and azathioprine) that dampen immune-mediated inflammatory reactions.

2. *"Is my family in danger, either by contagion or heredity?"* There is no scientific evidence to prove that IBD is contagious. Occasional clusters of cases by time and neighborhood have been found, but not often enough to support theories of infection. Likewise, cases have been reported in husbands and wives, but the frequency has been insufficient to prove that these are anything more than chance occurrences.

The evidence in favor of heredity, however, is much stronger, as you will read in detail in Chapter 9. Although inheritance of IBD is not straightforward or predictable, as it is in hemophilia, cystic fibrosis, or Tay-Sachs disease, there is no doubt that cases occur in blood relatives of patients far more often than could possibly be accounted for by chance.

What are the implications for patients having children? Simply put, a parent with IBD has somewhere between 3 to 8 percent chance of having a child with IBD. To be sure, this risk is about 10 times higher than the random risk for someone without an affected parent, but the fact remains that the odds are still against a child of an IBD patient ever developing IBD. People with IBD should therefore not avoid having children simply for fear of transmitting the disease. On the other hand, the risk of a child developing Crohn's disease if *both* parents have Crohn's disease appears to be nearly 50 percent. At this level of risk, genetic considerations might more reasonably play a role in family planning decisions.

3. *"Is this a Jewish disease?"* Not any more. About 40 or 50 years ago, the IBD risk for Jews was nearly 10 times higher than for the non-Jewish population, but times have changed. While there still seems to be roughly a two-to-threefold increase in incidence among Jews, over the general population, the rates in recent years have risen so dramatically among non-Jews, including African-Americans and Hispanics, that the "Jewishness" of IBD may be a steadily receding phenomenon. Although IBD is relatively rare among Native Americans, Asians, and Black Africans, in most populations of the so-called developed world it is rapidly becoming an "equal opportunity disease."

4. *"Does diet have anything to do with IBD?"* Several studies have pointed to certain dietary patterns as increasing the risk of IBD. These suggested risk factors have included early introduction of cow's milk without breast feeding, high intake of sugar and other refined carbohydrates, and low-fiber diets. The influence of all these various dietary factors on the risk of developing IBD, however, appears so small that most experts in the field discount them as major possible causes of these diseases.

Certain dietary adjustments, as discussed in Chapter 15, may alleviate some of the symptoms of IBD, especially when the small bowel is severely narrowed or inflamed. However, no particular dietary precautions seem to cause or prevent a flare-up of IBD and no particular dietary regimen seems to cure it.

5. *"Does IBD have any influence on sex life?"* As a rule, people who are in constant pain or who are feeling generally ill are not going to experience their customary sex drive. Moreover, a number of women with Crohn's disease may suffer from vaginal complications, including fistulas and abscesses, that can make sexual intercourse uncomfortable if not downright impossible. Beyond these general principles and specific examples, however,

there isn't anything in the nature of IBD itself that should interfere with the satisfactory pursuit and enjoyment of sex.

The various medical and surgical treatments used for IBD are also generally without major impact on sexual function. This includes ostomy surgery as well. Sulfasalazine temporarily interferes with male fertility but has no effect on sexual drive or potency. A tiny proportion of men who undergo total proctocolectomy (removal of the entire colon and rectum) may suffer pelvic nerve damage that could cause impotence, but the frequency of this complication in simple colitis operations (as opposed to the more radical procedures involved in cancer surgery) is today close to zero. In any event, doctors and patients should really get used to talking more openly about the sexual impact of chronic illnesses, including IBD.

6. *"How can you tell the difference between ulcerative colitis and Crohn's disease, and which is better to have?"* If the disease affects any part of the small intestine, or if it creates any major problems with fistulas or abscesses around the rectum, then it is definitely Crohn's disease. If, however, it is strictly limited to the large intestine ("colitis"), then it could be either ulcerative colitis or Crohn's disease, but the distinction between them doesn't always make much difference. The medical treatment for the two conditions is virtually identical. The only differences are that metronidazole and "bowel rest" with intravenous feeding or total parenteral nutrition (TPN) are often useful treatments for Crohn's disease but never for uncomplicated ulcerative colitis. Otherwise the medications used and doses prescribed are almost exactly the same.

The only time it becomes absolutely critical to distinguish between the two diseases is when an operation is being planned. Sometimes partial resections of the colon are possible in Crohn's disease, with reconnection of normal or less affected parts. Such measures are almost never

Want to Feel "In Control?" Learn More about Your Disease

Several recent studies have found that disease-related information is valued by people with chronic illness, even though it does not necessarily lead to improved health. In a recent study of the unmet needs of 377 patients with lupus, 32 percent of patients identified the lack of disease information as a major problem. In a 1987 study of 80 IBD patients, 77 percent of the respondents felt they had too little information about their disease, and *no patient had too much information.* Interestingly, the primary source of disease information for 87 percent of the respondents in this study was the physician.

The value of disease-specific information to IBD patients was explored in a study by psychologists **Mary Ellen Olbrisch** and **Stan Ziegler.** In their study of members of CCFA's Houston Chapter, they found no relationship between the amount of disease-specific information a patient possessed and the usefulness of that information in helping with disease management. This finding was probably a reflection of the fact that flare-ups of IBD are often poorly controlled and cannot be prevented by available medications. However, these investigators found a significant positive relationship between the amount of IBD information people possessed and how useful they felt it was in adapting to the emotional stress of living with the disease. In other words, learning about IBD, while not contributing to *actual* control over symptoms, helped to impart a *feeling* of control over the illness, and better adjustment to it.

possible in ulcerative colitis, where definitive surgery invariably requires removal of the entire colon. In this respect, Crohn's disease might be considered "better."

On the other hand, there are the new pull-through operations for ulcerative colitis described in Chapter 7. These procedures cannot be performed for Crohn's disease, so in this respect ulcerative colitis might be considered "better." Most important, total removal of the colon and rectum with construction of an ileostomy is a cure for ulcerative colitis, while the same operation for Crohn's disease carries a small but measurable chance (about 20 percent) that the inflammation might recur in the remaining small intestine. In this respect too, ulcerative colitis might be considered "better."

On balance, there is little to choose between one disease or the other. Which one is "better" depends upon how serious each particular case or its complications happen to be. Besides, the question of choice is essentially pointless to begin with; people don't get to choose their disease and they must cope with whatever it is they have.

7. *"Could I suffer any permanent ill effects from my medications?"* Most of the drugs commonly prescribed for IBD have been around so long that their track records are already pretty well known. These medications probably carry no hidden "time bombs" that will explode unexpectedly years later. Moreover, even the worst of the acute reactions caused by these drugs are usually temporary. The male infertility induced by sulfasalazine, the terrible cosmetic and psychological effects of steroids, the acute pancreatitis that may occur in 3 to 4 percent of patients on immunosuppressives, and the allergic fevers or rashes that some of these drugs may precipitate—all are ultimately reversible when the drugs are stopped. The numbness and tingling in the extremities that metronidazole (Flagyl®) often produces is

also usually reversible, although rare cases have persisted for many months or even years.

There are, however, several side effects of steroids that may be permanent and even disabling. One such side effect is cataracts, which may develop quite rapidly on long-term steroids. Even more serious, perhaps because they are not easily corrected, are the crippling effects that long-term high-dose steroids may have on bones. **Osteoporosis** (a thinning of bone tissue) is a risk for anyone on long-term steroids, especially postmenopausal women, who are particularly susceptible to collapsed vertebrae and other fractures. An even more devastating skeletal complication of long-term steroid treatment is **aseptic necrosis** of the hips, in which one or both hip joints may suddenly and without warning undergo massive deterioration. Men and women of all ages must be alert to this danger if they are being treated with high doses of corticosteroid drugs like prednisone for prolonged periods of time.

About 70 to 75 percent of people with Crohn's disease undergo surgery at some point in their illness, and virtually all of them are better off for having done so.

---

8. *"I've heard you should never operate on Crohn's disease because it always comes back again."* You've heard wrong. An operation is very often the best treatment for Crohn's disease. In fact, about 70 to 75 percent of people with Crohn's disease undergo surgery at some point in their illness, and virtually all of them are better off for having done so.

You've also heard right, at least to some extent. Surgery does *not* permanently cure

Crohn's disease. If it did, people would be operated on as soon as the diagnosis was made and would never have to deal with the disease again. Matters are obviously not that simple; after surgery, the disease tends to recur. But let's look more closely at what that means.

When we say Crohn's disease "recurs," that can mean at least three different things. First, it can mean that if we examine the site of previous surgery through an endoscope a year later, and if we take biopsies and scrutinize the tissues under a microscope, we find inflamed cells at least 90 percent of the time. But people don't usually care whether or not some tiny abnormalities show up under a microscope; they care about whether they will have symptoms or feel well.

The issue of having symptoms brings us to a second way of looking at postoperative "recurrence": Will the patient get *sick* again? Here the situation is not so bleak. Each year after surgery, only about 10 percent of postoperative patients will experience a symptomatic relapse, and these symptoms may respond better to standard medical therapies than the original condition did before surgery became necessary.

---

*Surgery does not represent
some kind of failure,
some sort of desperate measure,
a sentence of doom.
Surgery is just one more form
of treatment for Crohn's disease.*

There is also a third way of looking at the problem of recurrence: What are the chances someone will need *another* operation? The figures are relatively straightforward on this subject. Fewer than half the people who undergo routine surgery

for Crohn's disease—approximately 45 percent will someday need a second operation, usually 5 to 10 years later. And what about everybody's nightmare of needing one operation after another until there is no more intestine left to live on? The simple fact is that when someone undergoes a first operation for Crohn's disease, that person has only about one chance in ten of ever needing two or more subsequent operations throughout the rest of his/her life.

It is very important to keep the issue of surgery in perspective. Surgery does not represent some kind of failure, some sort of desperate measure, a sentence of doom. Surgery is just one more form of treatment for Crohn's disease. After all, the whole point of treatment is not the avoidance of surgery. The primary goal is *to be well.* If that goal can be achieved safely and successfully without an operation, so much the better. We'd all rather be kept feeling well by taking a few pills than by having an operation! But if having an operation is what it takes to be well, to be put back on our feet so that we can lead normal lives again, then we shouldn't be afraid of it; we should welcome it.

9. *"Is it true that nobody dies of Crohn's disease?"* Of course not. But that's the wrong question. Everybody dies of something. The question is not whether Crohn's disease is ever a cause of death; the question is whether Crohn's disease is a cause of *premature* death. In other words, is it likely to be responsible for a shortened life span? The answer is only very slightly if at all. Suppose, for example, that we take 100 people with Crohn's disease, and another 100 people of the same sex and age without Crohn's disease, and we follow both groups for the next 20 years. Statistics show that perhaps two people from the non-Crohn's group will die compared to about four people from the Crohn's group. Looking at these figures, an alarmist might say that Crohn's disease is responsible for a

doubling of the mortality rate. Looking at the same figures, however, a practical person would correctly conclude that Crohn's disease is responsible for no more than an extra 2 percent mortality.

What is the source of this extra 2 percent mortality rate among people with Crohn's disease? More than 20 years ago, the causes of these extra deaths were most often postoperative complications, infections, malnutrition, and a rare infection-related disorder called amyloidosis. In recent years, however, the picture has changed as these complications have been largely controlled or eliminated. Currently, the principal cause of Crohn's disease-related death is gastrointestinal cancer. In fact, physicians and patients are gradually coming to the realization that very longstanding Crohn's disease, especially when it involves a broad extent of colon, carries an increased risk of cancer similar to the well-recognized risk in ulcerative colitis. With heightened surveillance for early warning signs of malignant cells, the increased cancer risks and related mortality rates for both types of IBD should be substantially improved in the years ahead.

10. *"Does everyone with ulcerative colitis eventually develop colon cancer"?* Definitely not! After the first ten years of extensive disease, perhaps only 0.5 to 1 percent of ulcerative colitis patients ever develop cancer annually. Remember, too, that about 20 percent of those with extensive ulcerative colitis eventually undergo colectomy, effectively removing their risk altogether. The bottom line is that fewer than 5 percent of all people with ulcerative colitis will ever develop colon cancer at any time in their lives.

Today, most gastroenterologists recommend periodic surveillance (usually every one to two years) with colonoscopy and multiple biopsies (tissue samples) of the colon lining. During colonoscopic examination, the physician is able to look for any lesions along the whole length of the colon that might be cancerous or precancerous. Tissue samples taken during biopsy are examined carefully by a pathologist for signs of **dysplasia** (early pre-malignant cell changes). When dysplasia is found, there is approximately a 50 percent chance that cancer is already present somewhere in the colon; the earlier the dysplasia is detected, the lower the likelihood of there already being co-existing cancer. Therefore, most gastroenterologists consider dysplasia to be an absolute indication for colectomy. If colon cancer is not widespread when first diagnosed, the outlook for survival is excellent.

Part Two: Understanding IBD Treatments

Part III

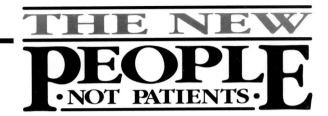

**THE NEW
PEOPLE
·NOT PATIENTS·**

IBD and the Life Cycle

Genetics and IBD: What We Know, What We Don't Know

9

Questions about the role genetic factors play in inflammatory bowel disease arise in several important situations. They can occur to the parents of a child with IBD, who might wonder what the risks are that their other children will develop IBD. Questions about genetics also are raised by couples contemplating childbearing, where one member (or rarely both) of the couple has IBD, or when the couple is already expecting a child. They can occur even earlier, when couples are contemplating solidifying their relationship through marriage and childbirth, and want to make their decisions in an informed manner. And finally, the question of genetic factors in IBD frequently comes up when anyone affected with IBD simply asks the question: "Why me, why did I get this disease?"

This chapter will summarize briefly what is known about the inheritance of IBD and the importance of genetic factors. It will also include what the actual risks are to family members, and how we counsel families with IBD regarding such risks.

The single greatest and best-established risk factor for developing IBD is a positive family history.

The most important point is that the accumulation of a large body of scientific evidence *does* indicate that genetic factors are of major importance in determining who in a population or in a family develops IBD. The single greatest and best-established risk factor for developing IBD is a positive family history, that is, having one or more relatives with IBD. A positive family history for IBD clearly and unequivocally increases one's risk, and is much better established as a risk factor than any other proposed risk factors such as diet, use of oral contraceptives, smoking, breast feeding, or any other life style or environmental factors. In fact, the risk for IBD to a first-degree relative (parent, brother, sister, or child) of an IBD patient is about 30 times greater than the risk to the general population. However, it is important to put this number in perspective. The average *actual* risk to brothers and sisters of an IBD patient obtained from several studies is approximately 2 to 6 percent. The risk to children may be as high, and that to parents may be slightly less. While the risk is much higher than it is for the general population, it still means that most of the relatives of an IBD patient will never develop IBD. Just as important, it also means that most people with IBD do *not* have an affected relative. Among patients with IBD, some 10 to 20 percent will report that another relative is affected. While this is much greater than the general population, still the majority of patients do not have a positive family history.

Heredity vs. Environment

Is this increased risk for family members entirely the result of genetic factors? After all, families don't share only their genes; they share their environment, where they live, what they eat, what viruses or other infectious agents they are exposed to. How do we know that the increased familial risk is due to genetic rather than environmental factors? We know this from two lines of evidence. One is from observing the frequency of IBD amoung the spouses of IBD patients. Husbands and wives of individuals with IBD clearly share much the same environment—they live in the same household, they eat many of the same foods. If local environment were extremely important to the development of IBD, we would expect spouses to have an increased frequency of the disease. All the available data indicate that spouses do *not* appear to be at higher risk, supporting the concept that the increased familial risk for IBD is due to genetic rather than environmental factors.

A second line of evidence comes from studies of twins. These studies are especially interesting because they provide a type of control for environmental exposure. Clearly, twins tend to share the same environment, at least throughout childhood. There are two kinds of twins. Identical or **monozygotic** twins arise from a single fertilized egg. They therefore share all their genes in common. Fraternal, nonidentical, or **dizygotic** twins occur from two different eggs, each fertilized by a different sperm. Therefore, fraternal twins have the same genetic resemblance as any pair of siblings (about half their genes in common). The only real difference between fraternal twins and siblings is that twins are raised together, and share their environment.

The way researchers use information on twins is to compare the **concordance** rates—that is the risk that the second twin is affected, between the twin pairs. If the identical and fraternal concordance rates are the same, this means that environmental factors determine the increased familial risk. Instead, what is observed in IBD is that the identical twin concordance rate is much higher than the fraternal rate (but even the identical twin concordance rate is not 100 percent). This tells us that the familial risk for IBD is due in large measure to genetic factors. Studies of fraternal twins show us that their risk is about the same size as that for siblings. This suggests that if the environment is indeed important (which is suggested by the large geographic variation in frequency of IBD worldwide), the important environment factors are likely those that affect the *whole* population and differ between populations (such as the degree of water sanitation), rather than local environmental factors, such as individual diets, that vary greatly within a population.

There are more things we don't know than we do know about the genetics of IBD.

Even with this knowledge, there are more things we don't know than we do know about the genetics of IBD. We really *don't* know how IBD is inherited. It does appear from the data on families and twins that we are looking at inherited genetic susceptibility to environmental agents that are likely to be widely available in any one population. However, we don't know how that susceptibility is inherited. We do know that it is not inherited in what is termed a simple Mendelian fashion—that is, the susceptibility to IBD is not inherited in a dominant fashion like eye color, a recessive fashion like Tay-Sachs or sickle cell disease, nor is it sex-linked. We are not yet sure if we have identified any of the actual genes that predispose someone to develop IBD, although research in that area is increasingly active and of great importance. In fact, there is tentative and extremely suggestive information about certain genes on chromosome number 6, and certain abnormalities of intestinal permeability, colonic mucins, and certain autoantibodies in families with IBD. These findings are very exciting, but cannot yet be used to predict whether specific individuals will develop IBD.

IBD and Ethnicity

Just as the frequency of IBD varies among families, it also varies among ethnic groups and different populations throughout the world. IBD appears more frequently in developed versus underdeveloped societies. This difference seems to be real, even with the very obvious differences in access to medical care. Even within the developed world, however, there are geographic and other differences. The most consistent difference is that individuals of Jewish ancestry appear to be at two to three times higher risk for IBD than their non-Jewish neighbors. How much genetic versus environmental factors determine this difference is still being investigated. Of course, this risk is still much smaller than the risk to a relative of someone with IBD, regardless of whether that individual is Jewish or non-Jewish.

Finding the IBD Genes

Of what use would it be to actually identify the genes for IBD? There are several reasons why it is extremely important for the medical research and IBD communities to support efforts to identify the actual genes for IBD. First, identifying these genes will allow the study of their structure and function, giving us a much better understanding of the causes of IBD. Understanding the causes will lead to new and improved therapies. Second, identification of the genes for IBD

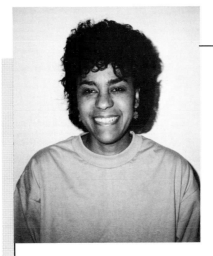

Martha Stone

Martha Stone is a sales professional at AT&T in her early forties who developed Crohn's disease over a decade ago. Her story is not unusual except that she is Black, and that two other family members—her sister, a cardiologist, and a niece (her brother's daughter) also have Crohn's disease. Diagnosed in her early 30's after several obstructive episodes and surgery for a rectal fistula, Martha feels that her diagnosis—and her sister's—would have been made years earlier had her doctors considered Blacks at risk for IBD. Although IBD has been considered more common in whites, recent studies from Baltimore show a rising trend among Blacks, particularly Black women. For her, Martha says, "Being Black with IBD is no different from being white or any other race. This disease doesn't discriminate."

Although she does not worry that her four year-old adopted son, Matthew will develop Crohn's disease, she is concerned that he has suffered as a result of her illness, particularly during her most recent hospitalization and recovery from surgery. When he can't find her, Martha says, her son has already learned to look first in the bathroom.

will provide the tools for better genetic counseling. Third, and potentially very exciting, identification of the IBD genes will enable us to identify people who are at a high risk for developing the disease. Study of these individuals will allow us to understand the process that converts genetic susceptibility into actual clinical disease, and eventually will lead to methods of disease prevention in these high risk individuals.

Genetic Counseling Advice for the Family with IBD

What genetic counseling advice do we give individuals with IBD and their families today? There are three major lessons. First it is important to emphasize that with our current understanding, the principal reason anyone has IBD is simply bad luck: that person received a combination of genes from either (or likely both) of their parents predisposing him/her to develop IBD. There is nothing known that a parent could have done that either led to a child having IBD or could have prevented it. Second, either form of IBD—ulcerative colitis or Crohn's disease—can occur in a family. The clinical form of IBD does not necessarily breed true. Third, and most important, even though the risk for IBD to family members is much greater than the general population, in terms of genetic risks it is still relatively small. If we take as an estimate that the risk to offspring for IBD is 5 percent (and it may be lower), that risk is 1 in 20. Such a risk also means that 19 out of 20 (or 95 percent) of children in a family with IBD will *not* have IBD. It is extremely important that these risks be placed in the proper perspective, since a number of families have the mistaken impression that the risk of a child developing IBD is overwhelming. Clearly the vast majority of relatives of an IBD patient will never develop IBD. It is a long term goal of genetic research in IBD to prevent this risk altogether.

Your Child with IBD—
A Guide for Parents

10

It is not easy sitting across from your child's doctor and being told that your child has a chronic illness for which there is no cure. The doctor reassures you that the overwhelming majority of kids actually do quite well, go to school, and do all the things that other kids do. But you do not hear that part. You only hear the words ulcerative colitis or Crohn's disease and you think the worst. You think that this newly diagnosed illness will be a threat to your child's development, happiness, and possibly even his/her life. This is when you need to take a big breath and *try* once again to listen to the doctor's words. This is the time that you need to find out what needs to be done now to make your child well again. It is also the time when you need to become *accurately* informed about your child's illness. The more you understand about IBD, the more skillful you will be in aiding your child and family in dealing with the illness.

Why My Child?

Despite many years of intensive research, we still do not know the exact cause or causes of IBD. There is a great deal of information suggesting that the body's immune system plays an important role in IBD. It is possible the immune system is attacking the intestinal tract. It is also possible, but not certain, that an infection or an allergy may trigger this attack. Heredity seems to be important and IBD does run in certain families. One thing we are sure of is that, as a parent, there is *nothing* that you *did* or *did not do* to cause IBD in your child.

When one child is diagnosed with Crohn's disease or ulcerative colitis, many parents worry that their other children may develop the disease. Be reassured that the risk of another child developing IBD is actually relatively small (See Chapter 9). It is estimated that about 2 to 6 percent of siblings may develop IBD during their lifetime. In other words, there is about a 95 percent chance that your other children will not develop IBD.

Between Onset and Diagnosis

As you have read in Chapter 2, it may take some time before the diagnosis of IBD can be made and treatment can be started. The length of time between the onset of symptoms and diagnosis in IBD varies greatly from one person to another. In children and adolescents, it is not unusual to wait 6 to 18 months before learning that your child has Crohn's disease or ulcerative colitis. This is because so many of the symptoms such as fatigue, loose stools, and abdominal pain, are **non-specific.** This means that they can be caused by many conditions, including irritable bowel syndrome (IBS), or by stress and anxiety. Even the passage of small amounts of blood in the stool may be interpreted as local irritation or the result of a hemorrhoid.

You need to know that a delay in diagnosis is unlikely to have any long-term consequences for your child.

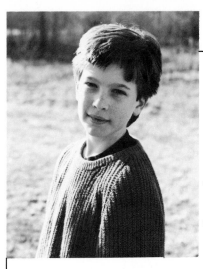

Josh Jubelirer

Josh Jubelirer, age 12, has had Crohn's disease since the age of five but you wouldn't know it to look at him. According to his mother, Shelly, an art teacher in Milwaukee where the Jubelirer family lives, "baseball is Josh's life!" In fact, last summer he only missed one game and that was because of a bout with asthma, not Crohn's disease.

Josh's parents have encouraged him to take charge of his treatments—although he does get an occasional unsolicited reminder to take his medicines from his two brothers and his sister. Thanks to his mother, Josh's teachers know about his illness and that he may have to leave the classroom to use the bathroom. With a support system at home and at school, Josh can feel "in charge."

Many parents worry that a delay in diagnosis—and a corresponding delay in treatment—will mean that the IBD will be more severe as a result. You need to know that a delay in diagnosis is unlikely to have any long-term consequences for your child. You and your child's physician need to start thinking about what needs to be done *now*, not what might have been done one year ago.

Telling Your Child about IBD

Children fantasize about illness and often the fantasy is much more frightening than the reality. They will look to their parents for clues about how they should feel and act. You should be reassuring in your approach and should not try to hide information if your child asks for it. At the same time, it is important to recognize that very young children may be limited in their ability to understand everything that we tell them. Your child's physician—and your common sense—will help you to know what your child is prepared to hear and understand.

In explaining about the disease, you can tell your child that the doctor has said that the intestine is inflamed. This means that it is red, swollen, and tender, much like a child's knee immediately after a scrape. This inflammation causes the bleeding, cramps, and loss of appetite that your child has experienced. Fortunately, you can tell your child that there are medicines that can relieve this inflammation.

It is also likely that your child will need many tests—such as blood tests, x-rays, and endoscopy or sigmoidoscopy—to establish the diagnosis of IBD. While these tests may be uncomfortable and a bit frightening, they help the physician to localize the inflammation and to decide exactly which medications are most suitable to treat your child. In addition, blood tests are usually necessary periodically to assess the activity of disease and to watch for any important side-effects of medications. Blood tests are frightening to children—and to many adults, too. You can help by reassuring your child that the results of these blood tests will allow the doctor to do an even better job in treating the inflammation.

Delayed Growth and IBD

About 30 percent of children with Crohn's disease and 10 percent of children with ulcerative colitis will experience some slowing of the growth process because of their illness. Most of the time, this delay in growth is caused by chronically poor nutrition (often the result of lack of appetite or abdominal pain) and the need for prolonged use of prednisone, a corticosteroid medication. (See Chapter 5 for an explanation of medications prescribed in IBD.) Your child's doctor will try to institute a program of nutritional supplementation, if necessary, and will try to keep the use of growth-retarding medications to a minimum (See below). There are times when your doctor may recommend surgery as the most appropriate way to treat both the IBD and the delay in growth.

IBD Medications in Children

The medications used to treat IBD in children are the same as those used for adults. Obviously, the medications are given in lower doses, depending on the age and weight of your child (See Chapter 5). Azulfidine® (sulfalalazine) and prednisone are the two most commonly used medications for both forms of IBD. Each has the ability to reduce inflammation in the affected intestine. Azulfidine,® which has a sulfa component as well as a part which resembles aspirin, is useful for mild to moderate inflammation of the colon. While it can sometimes cause nausea, abdominal

How to Explain IBD to Your Child

Explaining a serious illness to a young child is a difficult and painful task. **Mary-Joan Gerson, Ph.D.,** a psychologist on the faculty of Mount Sinai School of Medicine, offers several suggestions to parents:

- **Use pictorial representations.** Because children have a strong visual sense, pictures and diagrams help to clarify difficult subject matter. You might show your child a diagram of the gastrointestinal tract and explain in simple terms, how it works and what has gone wrong (See Chapter 1 of this book). During your discussion, the most important thing is to follow the cues of your child.
- **Encourage your child to write down his/her questions.** Often, when children are feeling anxious, they forget what they are told. Give your child a small blackboard or notebook to write down any questions. Later, he/she can discuss these issues with you and with the physician.
- **Proper preparation is essential.** Children with IBD undergo many uncomfortable gastrointestinal examinations. Many youngsters will require surgery. Fear of the unknown is a normal reaction. You can relieve some of your child's anxiety by explaining what will happen during a particular procedure. Before the discussion, review the information with the physician. Be sure that you understand it completely. This is important not only for your own peace of mind, but for that of your child.
- **Don't overwhelm your child with details.** Give him/her a basic outline of the medical problem or surgical procedure. Consider your child's level of understanding, personality, and attention span. Try to remember how you prepared your child for first grade or for camp. Being very concrete provides reassurance: "This is what will happen. I will be there when you come back from surgery. I will be there when you cry or are in pain."

pain, or headache, these side-effects generally lessen over the first week or two of treatment. Sometimes children develop a rash and the drug must be stopped; however, it frequently can be restarted in a very low dose which is then increased gradually. Newer medications (5-ASA agents) are now available which are similar to sulfasalazine but cause fewer allergic problems.

Prednisone, a potent anti-inflammatory medication, is used when the inflammation is located primarily in the small intestine or when the large intestine is severely inflamed. While prednisone is a very good drug for this purpose, it can cause problems that are particularly distressing to children and adolescents. These include puffiness around the face, increased body hair, acne, and red stretch marks on the abdomen. Since prednisone also causes the body to retain salt and water, your doctor may tell you to be careful about how much salt your child consumes (See Chapter 15). Avoiding foods like potato chips, pretzels, cold cuts and many junk foods will reduce the swelling caused by prednisone. You can reassure your child or teenager that the unpleasant side effects of prednisone will lessen and disappear completely when the drug is tapered and stopped.

As children get older, they should be encouraged to assume more responsibility for taking their medications.

It is very important that careful monitoring take place to ensure that medications are taken as prescribed. Children and adolescents sometimes stop taking their medications because of some of these side-effects. This may not only worsen the symptoms of IBD but may have other serious metabolic consequences for the body as well. Your child's doctor is also eager to taper the dosage of medications but this needs to be done in a controlled manner so that symptoms do not recur. At times, other medications, such as antibiotics or immunosuppressive agents like 6-mercaptopurine, may be used in conjunction with other therapy (See Chapter 5). Careful monitoring of blood counts and special biochemical tests are necessary when these medications are used.

Taking Medications: Whose Responsibility Is It?

With very young children, it is obvious that parents need to take the primary responsibility for providing medications at the correct times and in the correct doses. As children get older, they should be encouraged to assume more responsibility for taking their medications. However, because it is so important that medications are on schedule, parents of older children and adolescents often need to strike a difficult balance between being concerned and seeming unconcerned. This is much easier said than done!

The Importance of Good Nutrition

Nutritional therapy is an important part of your child's treatment. Fortunately, many children start to eat better as their gastrointesinal symptoms lessen. Prednisone itself seems to stimulate the appetite. Your child's doctor and dietician can suggest which foods to avoid during flare-ups; these include high fiber foods and milk products. In general, children with IBD should be encouraged to eat *what* they like and *when* they like. Even reasonable amounts of "junk food" are allowed (See Chapter 15).

Although it's a good idea to encourage your child to eat, you need to be careful not to make an issue of it. Loss of appetite is usually a part of the disease process, and not something that most children can easily control.

Occasionally, your child's appetite will not improve with medical therapy, and nutritional treatments may be necessary. Liquid supplements are available to add to the calories and nutrients taken with meals. (Chapter 16 contains a complete lisiting of these products.) At times these supplements must be given through a small soft tube which is placed through the nose into the stomach (nasogastric tube). This type of feeding usually starts shortly before bedtime and continues through the night. The tube is removed in the morning before school. Although this sounds frightening, most young people can learn to insert the tube and remove it themselves with little help. The increase in weight and improvements in appearance and energy over the first couple of weeks serve as excellent positive reinforcement for this form of treatment. If your child is taking prednisone, this type of intensive nutritional therapy often allows the doctor to taper the dose of prednisone even more quickly.

When Hospitalization Becomes Necessary

At times your child's illness may not respond to oral medications and nutritional therapy provided at home. Your doctor may tell you that your child needs intravenous medications, intravenous nutrition, and bowel rest in the hospital. In some cases, surgery may even be considered. Again, you will need to explain carefully to your child why the hospitalization is taking place and that stronger medications are needed to control symptoms. If surgery is required,

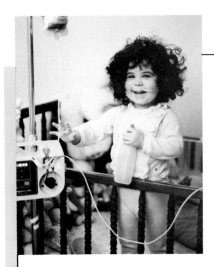

Elizabeth Wachstein

The feeding tube you see in this photograph is helping Elizabeth Wachstein, now age six, to get enough calories to grow normally. When this photo was taken, Elizabeth had already had Crohn's disease for four years; because the disease slowed her growth, tube feeding was started when she was two years old. Tube feeding takes away some of the worry parents have about providing enough nourishment for children with Crohn's disease who, like Elizabeth, often eat poorly.

Elizabeth goes to school with the tube in place, enjoys normal activities, and every two weeks assists her parents, Alison and Bob Wachstein of Weston, Connecticut, in changing the tubing. All this is not easy. Says Alison Wachstein, "The support of other mothers of children with IBD has helped me enormously."

All in the Family: Stresses and Strains Caused by IBD

The families of children with chronic illness share many common problems. These include overprotectiveness, overinvolvement of the family with the child's illness, isolation of the child from his/her siblings and peers, and avoidance of healthy expressions of anger and emotion.

In a recent CCFA study, the families of youngsters with Crohn's disease functioned less well psychologically than the families of children with ulcerative colitis. The authors speculate that because Crohn's disease is incurable, the prospect of recurrence and multiple surgery places enormous pressure on these children and their families.

Adjusting to Life with IBD

Families can overcome some of these pressures by being aware of potential problems, addressing them as they arise, if necessary, and seeking professional help. As much as possible considering the child's age, comprehension, and emotional development, he/she should begin to take over responsibility for managing the illness. It is understandable that parents, out of concern for the youngster's well-being, should find it difficult to relinquish responsiblity. But children who assume greater control of their own care as they grow older gain independence and greater self-confidence.

Families should strive to make the sick child feel that he/she is "just one of the family." "There are two things parents have to be careful about," cautions psychologist **Dr. Mary-Joan Gerson.** "In a two-parent home, the parents should collaborate in caring for the child. Otherwise, one parent becomes extra-involved. Also, the child with IBD tends to become isolated from his siblings. Though it's asking families already burdened with problems to do even more, they should make every effort to involve the sick child as much as possible with the day-to-day activities of the family."

(Continued on next page)

a diagram of the intestine is very helpful in pointing out to your child exactly what is going to be done. (Such a diagram appears in Chapter 1 of this book and can be filled in with the physician's help.) You can ask your child's physician or local chapter of CCFA or The United Ostomy Association (UOA) to locate another child of the same sex and age who has undergone a similar procedure. There is something very reassuring about having another 14 year-old tell your 14 year-old about "the operation" and how well he/she now feels. If your child is able to do schoolwork in the hospital, a couple of hours each day should be set aside for this purpose.

Telling Family, Friends and Your Child's School

Family and friends will frequently seek out information about your child's illness in order to be helpful. The amount of information that you share with them is entirely up to you and your child. Friends and relatives may offer well-meaning advice concerning the disease, its treatment, diet, stress, etc. Remember to put into perspective the anecdotal stories that are offered, especially if they describe someone with IBD who had either a difficult time or a "miracle cure." No two cases of IBD are alike and each requires an individual approach to treatment. Above all, ignore suggestions that your child has developed IBD as a result of stress. This is simply not true.

No child with IBD should be placed in an embarrassing situation because of the need to use a bathroom.

Informing your child's school about the diagnosis is very important for several reasons. Most importantly, your child may need to make frequent use of a bathroom when IBD is active. Using the bathroom frequently in school may be viewed by teachers as a way of avoiding classroom activities or engaging in smoking or even drug use. Unless the teacher and school nurse are aware of your child's needs, problems may arise. If possible, your child should be allowed free access to a teacher's bathroom or a bathroom located in the nurse's office. However, some young people with IBD choose not to be singled out in this way and prefer to use regular bathrooms. At the very least, no child with IBD should be placed in an embarrassing situation because of the need to use a bathroom.

At times participation in sports may be somewhat more difficult and allowances will have to be made. Medications may need to be given in school. To help school personnel understand and address your child's needs, ask your doctor to make up a package of educational pamphlets and bring them in yourself. CCFA publishes many informational brochures, including one for teachers. Have the nurse or teacher contact your child's doctor if there are any questions about medication or nutrition you feel unsure about answering.

IBD and Your Child's Future

None of us can predict the future, particularly for any one child. What we *can* tell you is that IBD is extremely unlikely to shorten your child's life. There will be hospitalizations and perhaps even surgery, but the good times will far outnumber the bad. For some children, there may be a delay in the onset of puberty but with appropriate treatment, development will proceed and be completed normally. Newer surgical methods have been developed that make it unnecessary to have a permanent ileostomy, should surgery be needed for the child with ulcerative colitis. (See Chapter 7).

(Continued from previous page)

The Pressure on Siblings

The brothers and sisters of a youngster with IBD often feel neglected. Encouraging your sick child to join in the family's activities enables you to spend more time with *all* of your children. You also can minimize resentment by having your child with IBD follow the family's rules regarding bedtime, allowances, and household chores.

Unfortunately, families of chronically ill children tend to avoid open confrontation. "This is probably because they must contend with so many crises and emergencies," says Dr. Gerson. "These families must learn to tolerate open conflict so the children—and the parents—can express anger openly. It's better for a sibling to say, 'I hate you because Daddy always drives you to the doctor,' than for him to store up this resentment."

(continued on next page)

(Continued from previous page)

Danger Signals

Most chronically ill children and their families learn to cope well. Sometimes, however, the pressures of the illness become too great for a child to handle. According to Dr. Gerson, the signs that a child requires professional counseling are:

- social isolation and depression
- boredom or listlessness
- lack of interest in relationships
- immature behavior not explained by illness

Of course, seriously ill children will go through periods when they don't feel well enough to take part in social activities. They may feel depressed or behave childishly to get attention from their parents. But if this behavior is prolonged, psychological counseling should be sought.

A child's inability to cope with the illness often is a sign that the family is undergoing a similar struggle. Thus, Dr. Gerson recommends a consultation for the entire family as a first step. "Too often, children are referred to individual therapists as if the problem were theirs alone—to figure out and to fix. Family therapists explore untapped resources in the family for coping with stress, at the same time that they address wider issues. Our preference is that family therapy be the initial treatment of choice."

If at all possible, your child's IBD should not become the focus of family life. Concessions will occasionally have to be made to the illness but every effort should be made to lead a normal family life. If discipline is required in a particular situation, it should be carried out appropriately. Along with medications, reassurance, love, and understanding are all important in helping your child become well again.

Managing IBD at College 11

Going off to college usually causes a variety of stresses for both parents and young people. Parents recognize that the time has come for their child to separate and become independent; "letting go" is not an easy task for parents. At the same time, while most teenagers look forward eagerly to being on their own, they may still have fears about entering new situations and separating completely from their parents. Imagine, in this situation, the added anxiety of having to deal with a chronic illness like inflammatory bowel disease!

If you are a young person with IBD going off to college, these are some of the questions you might have: Can your physician make this transition easier for you and your family? What issues should be discussed, and when? Should you select a school because it is near a good medical center? Should you choose a school close to home? Or should IBD have nothing to do with your choice of college? What happens when you have a flare-up or need to be hospitalized? There are no uniform answers to these questions.

Obviously, your choice of a college may be influenced by many factors, including whether you have mild or severe disease, an ostomy, or if you are receiving supplemental nutrition. It is reassuring to know that in most cases, although your time schedule may have to be modified somewhat, you can attend the college of your choice. No matter what school you select, adequate acute emergency care is almost always available through the student health services. It is always a good idea to familiarize the physicians and health personnel at your school with your case. Your physician will be happy to write and/or phone to explain your history and treatment. Attach your doctor's business card to your health form so communication is possible both day and night. You might also ask your doctor to recommend the name of a gastroenterologist knowledgeable about IBD in your college town. However it is important to know that your doctor can continue to care for you and manage your IBD even though you are away from home.

Quality of Life at College

Once you arrive at school, the availability of appropriate bathroom facilities may be of paramount concern to you. Some dormitories offer single rooms with a private bathroom, but most often bathrooms are shared by several students. You might want to inquire whether the bathrooms are shared by men and women. Are there enough toilet facilities and are the toilets themselves private? How far are the toilets from your room? Are there any bathroom facilities on the way to class? Are they open for use at all hours? Are there adequate bathroom facilities in the classroom buildings themselves? Do not be afraid to ask the school authorities any of these questions. Knowing the answers will make your life at school a lot less stressful.

You may also have specific concerns about the food at school. After all, your family has been cooking foods you like and can eat for some time. The fact is that most patients with IBD do not need to be on restricted diets. Young people with Crohn's disease and strictures may be on low fiber diets, but high fiber foods can easily be eliminated without avoiding the dining hall altogether. Avoid only those foods that are bothersome to you and try to maintain a weight agreed upon by you and your doctor.

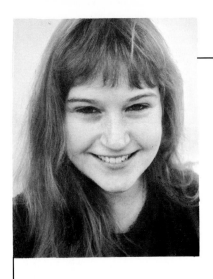

Netania Steiner

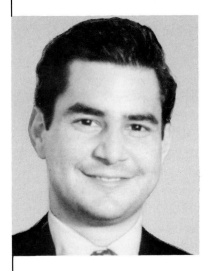

and Eric Wasserman

Long lines in the dining hall, a sprawling campus, and crowded parties with limited access to bathrooms are just a few of the problems students with IBD must face in going away to college. But for Netania Steiner and Eric Wasserman, leaving home was never in doubt. Now in their mid-twenties, both have some perspective on the college years.

"It was important for me to go away," says Steiner, a recent graduate of Wesleyan University, who now lives in New York City. "I didn't want to take the safe way out and I've gained so much self-confidence because of it."

But for Wasserman, who grew up in Florida and graduated a few years ago from Duke University, "having IBD never entered the decision-making process. It was never a cause for concern."

(continued on next page)

What if you are receiving nutritional supplements, either by nasogastric tube or intravenous infusion (TPN)? Your physician may be able to set up a working relationship between you and a nutritional support service in your college town. Most nutritional home care companies are capable of servicing any college population. If this is not possible, the local hospital may have a nutritional support program that can serve your needs. How you schedule your supplemental feedings should be flexible enough so that you can still enjoy college life. Check with your doctor to see what routine will allow you to achieve the desired caloric intake while imposing the least burden on your academic and social life.

Keeping Up with Your Studies

The academic demands on you will vary depending on the school you choose, your major, your study habits, and how well you feel. If getting out to class in the morning is a problem, try to arrange a schedule with no early morning classes. It is also good to remember that there is no law requiring that you graduate in four years. Many students take five or more years to graduate for lots of reasons other than IBD! You might want to check whether your college has a program through which you can recover partial or full tuition payments if you have to leave school for an extended period of time. Taking a slightly less demanding academic load may be preferable, especially when your disease is active.

Many students take five or more years to graduate for lots of reasons other than IBD!

If your school offers a study program abroad, don't let the fact that you have IBD prevent you from exploring this opportunity. There are gastroenterologists in most developed countries who can communicate with your doctor at home if the need arises. Usually, a few telephone calls will suffice to get you through a rough period.

Despite your busy schedule, you should make plans to see your physician at home at least once each year. This will give the two of you a chance to catch up on how you are doing medically and socially. You may also use these opportunities to discuss your plans for work, relocation to another part of the country, marriage and children. If you are on medication, you probably will need some routine blood work. Perhaps your medications should be altered or even discontinued if you have been in good health. Only by maintaining regular communication with your doctor can these important issues be discussed.

(continued from previous page)

Administrative vs. Social Problems

There are more differences than similarities in these two young people's college experiences. Eric graduated on time and was in remission most of the time. Netania was forced to withdraw to undergo ileostomy surgery just after starting her freshman year. "That was a big setback, but it was also a turning point in a way," she says. "I fought hard to go to school and this was a test for me. I didn't want Crohn's to stop me from doing anything." She returned to school the following January.

Still there were problems. The school was insistent that she graduate on time and take a regular course load. After a two-year struggle, she finally secured open-ended status, and graduated in June of 1990 despite several flare-ups and stays in the hospital. "You have to demand that they deal with you and your rights," she says. "You can't just ask nicely." For her, earning her college degree was a symbol that she could be successful despite her illness.

Eric Wasserman did not face the same problems at Duke. Most of his troubles were social in nature. "My problem at school was having to get up and walk out twice per seminar to use the bathroom," he says. "It's embarrassing. You don't want to be noticed and then you have to apologize and explain to your professor."

The lack of privacy in the dormitory and sharing a bathroom with 20 other students was also a problem. "In the dorm, there was never any place I could crawl away to," says Eric about the times he would feel sick. "Everyone was very conscious of it. People want to know what the problem is but you don't want to be the topic of conversation. Sure, my close friends knew about it. They could check on me and they were people to talk to. Still, I tried to keep it quiet."

(continued on next page)

(continued from previous page)

Meeting the Challenge

Having IBD did not stop either student from accomplishing what they wanted to in college. Eric majored in public policy, served as vice president of his dorm, was active in intramural sports, and is now an equity research analyst for a brokerage firm in New York City. Netania majored in history, wrote a historical novel as her graduation thesis, and became a popular rock and blues singer on campus. She now works as a musician.

Both agree that you should try not to feel like a victim of IBD. "You can't let the disease control you," says Eric. Netania seconds the motion: "I think it would be a mistake for someone not to go away to school just because he or she has IBD. It's easy to fall into a safe, protective pattern. It's so easy to lose your independence, settle down, and give up your goals."

"I want this disease to be just a footnote in my life."

Pregnancy and IBD

12

Many women with Crohn's disease or ulcerative colitis are concerned about whether they will be able to become pregnant and whether their disease will affect the outcome of the pregnancy. There are also many questions and concerns about whether it is safe to use IBD medications before and during pregnancy. In this chapter, we will provide the latest information about these very important concerns.

Fertility and IBD

In general, women with Crohn's disease or ulcerative colitis whose disease is inactive have the same ability to conceive as do other women in the general population. Furthermore, women whose disease is under good control with medical treatment usually have no difficulty becoming pregnant. However, it is known that women with active Crohn's disease may be less able to become pregnant. There are several reasons why this is so. A major reason is that the active disease has resulted in poor nutrition. Another reason is that when Crohn's disease is very active in the small intestine, the inflammation may interfere with the function of the ovaries nearby and may cause some pelvic scarring. Abscesses and fistulas to and around the vagina may even interfere with sexual intercourse. Nevertheless, when Crohn's disease is brought under control with appropriate medications, the ability to conceive is almost always restored.

When IBD is under good control or even mildly active, there is no reason to fear becoming pregnant.

Some women with IBD are afraid to become pregnant for fear of having a complicated pregnancy or an abnormal baby. Occasionally, a physician may advise a woman not to become pregnant because of her IBD; unfortunately, this misinformation may cause some women to avoid pregnancy altogether. This is most unfortunate because when IBD is under good control or even mildly active, there is no reason to fear becoming pregnant. If there is active disease accompanied by significant abdominal pain and diarrhea, it is a good idea to wait until the disease has gone into remission or has improved significantly before becoming pregnant. Nevertheless, most women with IBD will be able to conceive and will experience a normal pregnancy.

The Effect of IBD on Pregnancy

Understandably, women are often concerned about whether inflammatory bowel disease will affect the outcome of the pregnancy. Fortunately, at least 80 percent of women with inactive IBD will experience a normal full-term delivery, much the same as women in the general population. However, for a woman with active IBD during pregnancy, there is a two to three times greater chance of spontaneous abortion and preterm birth. This is especially true for a woman who develops Crohn's disease during pregnancy. The important thing to remember is that the increased risk to the fetus is *not* the result of taking IBD medications but is caused by the activity of the disease itself. Therefore your gastroenterologist will advise you that if your disease is not active during pregnancy, you can look forward to giving birth to a healthy, full-term baby. However, if your

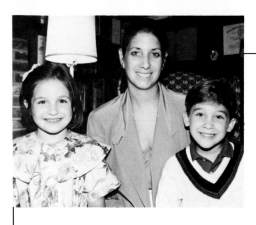

Valerie Morello

Valerie Morello's doctors told her that she was too sick to withstand the stress of pregnancy, so, reluctantly, she and her husband Michael, residents of Vineland, New Jersey, put off starting a family. Diagnosed with Crohn's disease when she was a college freshman, Valerie had spent the equivalent of two years in the hospital and almost three years on nasogastric tube feeding. "You wait for years to have a child," she says, "and then the disease forces you to change your plans." After surgery brought Valerie's disease into remission, the Morellos finally decided to adopt. Just 10 and a half months after welcoming their daughter, Danielle, in October of 1985, Valerie gave birth to their son, Matthew!

The pregnancy went extremely smoothly and Valerie has been without symptoms—and without medications— for over seven years now. A former president of CCFA's Philadelphia/Delaware Valley Chapter and former Northeast Regional President, Valerie is now in her second year at Rutgers University Law School. How does she feel about being told initially not to have children? "In a way, it turned out for the best, because otherwise we might never have adopted our wonderful daughter. But I would never advise any woman with IBD to avoid becoming pregnant just because of the disease. For me, pregnancy—and motherhood—have been wonderful experiences."

disease flares up during pregnancy, this does *not* mean that you cannot continue the pregnancy. It does mean that your gastroenterologist will recommend that you take medications to control the symptoms of IBD during your pregnancy (See below).

The Effect of Pregnancy on Disease Activity

Most women whose disease is inactive before pregnancy will stay in remission during pregnancy. However, active disease prior to pregnancy may actually get worse during the pregnancy. This usually happens during the first trimester, or at the end of the third trimester and during the postpartum period. Although there is no good explanation for a flare-up of IBD during the first trimester, a flare-up in the postpartum period may be the result of a decrease in the body's natural corticosteroid levels after delivery.

Approximately half of the women who have their initial episode of IBD during pregnancy will have severe disease. However, this is *not* a reason for a woman to undergo an abortion. With medical therapy, the symptoms of IBD often resolve and the pregnancy will continue normally.

In general, the course of IBD during pregnancy is no different than it is at other times. Activity of the disease during one pregnancy has no bearing on the course of future pregnancies.

Taking Medications during Pregnancy

Women often ask whether the medicines they take to control the symptoms of IBD will cause problems during pregnancy or cause harm to the fetus. Ideally, of course, it would be best for every pregnant woman to avoid medication during the full term of her pregnancy. However, more than three-quarters of women with IBD will be on some medication at the time they may consider having a child. Therefore, it is important to discuss the safety of current medical therapy and dispel some of the fears that might arise when your gastroenterologist suggests continuing your medication during pregnancy. Fortunately, the drugs used most often in treatment—sulfasalazine and cortisteroids—have proved to be extremely safe during pregnancy. The following section will discuss what is known about the safety during pregnancy of these and other medications currently used to treat IBD.

Sulfasalazine

It is theoretically possible for the sulfa part of sulfasalazine to cross the placenta and reach the fetus, resulting in jaundice (yellow skin and eyes in the fetus.) However, this complication is probably extremely rare and it has not been reported frequently in the medical literature. Sulfasalazine may also be present in breast milk but no complications have been reported in breast-fed infants. Therefore, experience over many years has shown that it is really quite safe for a woman to continue taking sulfasalazine during and after pregnancy. It is important to note that sulfasalazine does interfere with the absorption of folic acid, a vitamin important in cell growth and, therefore, in fetal development. Your obstetrician or gastroenterologist should make sure you are taking 1 mg of folic acid each day if you remain on sulfasalazine.

5-Aminosalicylic Acid (5-ASA)

Now that Dipentum,® the first oral 5-aminosalicylic acid compound, has been approved for the treatment of IBD, many of the concerns about the side effects of sulfasalazine are no longer relevant. This is because Dipentum® contains no sulfa, the substance responsible for most of the side effects of sulfasalazine treatment. However,

Infertility in Men with IBD

In men who have IBD, taking sulfasalazine can result in a decreased sperm count and decreased motility of the sperm. This effect on sperm occurs approximately two months after starting the drug; fortunately, infertility is reversed about two months after the drug is stopped. The good news is that this reversible abnormality appears to be caused by the sulfapyridine portion of the drug and *not* by 5-aminosalicylic acid, the active portion of sulfasalazine. The new salicylate preparations (e.g. Dipentum®) do not contain sulfapyridine.

In rare circumstances, men with IBD may be infertile because of an inability to have an erection following total proctocolectomy (removal of the colon and rectum). Another uncommon complication following surgery is retrograde ejaculation, in which the sperm are directed backward into the bladder. Fortunately, these complications of ileostomy surgery are both extremely rare.

because Dipentum® is so new, there are not enough studies to establish clearly its safety during pregnancy. It is a good idea to check with your gastroenterologist about the advisability of using this medication during pregnancy.

Corticosteroids

Corticosteroids (such as prednisone, Medrol,® ACTH, etc.) are known to cross the placenta and to cause prematurity, stillbirths and cleft palate in laboratory animals. However, this rarely happens in humans. It has been shown that prematurity and problems with the placenta occur much more frequently when a pregnant woman with active IBD is untreated. Therefore, there is a greater risk of *not treating* active IBD during pregnancy than there is in using steroids to treat active disease. The use of steroids while the mother is breast feeding is not known to cause any complications for the baby.

There is a greater risk of not treating *active IBD during pregnancy than there is in using steroids to treat active disease.*

Even though steroids are considered safe during pregnancy, most gastroenterologists recommend that they be discontinued during pregnancy if at all possible. However, if disease is active, it is still safer for the mother and fetus if the disease is treated with steroids because of the known risk to the fetus from active disease.

Metronidazole and Other Antibiotics

It is well known that metronidazole (Flagyl®) can cause tumors and other complications in laboratory animals. However, many women have been treated with short courses of metronidazole for vaginal infections without experiencing complications. Because the safety of this drug has not been established for long-term use during pregnancy, it should be avoided, especially during the first trimester. Metronidazole is found in the breast milk of nursing mothers. Since the potential side effects for the baby are not known, this drug should be avoided until after nursing is completed.

Other antibiotics have been used on occasion to treat mild IBD, especially Crohn's disease. However, these medications should not be used during pregnancy unless medically indicated, because *all* antibiotics appear in breast milk. It is not known whether they cause harm to the newborn and should be used only when prescribed by your doctor for a specific reason.

Immunosuppressive Agents— Azathioprine and 6-Mercaptopurine (6-MP)

Immunosuppressive agents, used most often to treat severe Crohn's disease, are known to be **teratogenic** in animals. That is, they are capable of causing deformities in the developing fetus. It is also true that in humans, normal infants have been born while the mother has been taking these agents for other serious illnesses, even in large doses. In a recent study of 14 women taking azathioprine during pregnancy, there were no congenital abnormalities or subsequent health problems in the newborns. The authors of this study concluded that termination of pregnancy is not required for women taking the drug during pregnancy. Another recent study reported that taking 6-MP before or at the time of conception did *not* increase the rate of spontaneous abortions or the number of birth defects in newborns.

Despite these encouraging studies, there are still concerns. Chief among these is the possible long-term genetic effect of immunosuppressives on the newborn. For this reason, immunosuppressive therapy should be used during pregnancy only if other medical therapies are not helping. If possible, immunosuppressives should be avoided during the first trimester of pregnancy, when the embryo is still developing. Nevertheless, most gastroenterologists still recommend that if a pregnancy is being planned, immunosuppressive therapy should be stopped before conception.

Alternative Treatment for IBD during Pregnancy

Occasionally, other methods of treatment have been used during pregnancy with beneficial results. **Total parenteral nutrition (TPN)** has been used instead of corticosteroids in some people, especially those with Crohn's disease. Unfortunately, there is not enough evidence that TPN is entirely safe during pregnancy; there is a possibility that this method of treatment may increase the formation of gallstones. A few studies have demonstrated a decrease in the symptoms of small bowel Crohn's disease using what is called an **elemental diet.** Elemental diets allow essential nutrients to be absorbed very easily by the inflamed intestine and cause very little residue. In some people, this alternative method of treatment has been as successful as steroids in decreasing the symptoms of Crohn's disease.

Chapters 15 and 16 contain important information about the role of good nutrition in the overall health of people with IBD. Obviously, despite the presence of IBD, it is extremely important for the mother and fetus to have an adequate nutritional and vitamin intake during the course of pregnancy.

Nutritional supportive therapy should be considered as adjunctive, or additional, therapy when appropriate. In general, it is a good idea to avoid antidiarrheal medications such as Imodium® and Lomotil,® especially during the first trimester of pregnancy. In particular, narcotic antidiarrheals, such as codeine and deodorized tincture of opium (DTO), should be avoided, because of the possibility that the newborn may become addicted to them.

Diagnostic Testing during Pregnancy

A few studies have shown that small amounts of radiation from x-rays have not been associated with any cancers or deformities in the newborn. Nevertheless, unless medically necessary, it is wise to avoid all x-ray studies during pregnancy, especially during the first trimester. If your gastroenterologist thinks it is necessary to determine disease activity or to make changes in therapy, it is considered safe to undergo flexible sigmoidoscopy with biopsy and, in rare cases, even colonoscopy and upper endoscopy.

Surgery and Pregnancy

If IBD is in remission or is well controlled during pregnancy, surgery is rarely necessary. In a few rare cases surgery may be required during pregnancy either for severe ulcerative colitis, toxic megacolon, or for obstruction or perforation of the bowel in Crohn's disease. When this happens, the fetus usually fares better if the surgery occurs later in pregnancy. However, if surgery is performed earlier in the course of pregnancy, spontaneous abortion or prematurity occurs in about 50 percent of cases.

The good news is that for the majority of women with IBD, a normal vaginal delivery is preferred unless there are obstetrical reasons to perform a caesarean section.

Women who have had previous surgery for IBD (resection, colectomy and ileostomy, continent ileostomy, or ileoanal anastomosis) often wonder whether they can have a normal delivery and whether caesarean section will be necessary. The good news is that for the majority of women with IBD, a normal vaginal delivery is preferred unless there are obstetrical reasons to perform a caesarean section. Only in women with severe perineal disease is caesarean delivery strongly recommended.

During the course of the pregnancy the enlarging abdomen may cause some problems with the size and contour of an ileostomy. If this happens, a larger appliance will often be necessary. Prolapse of the ileostomy may also occur, but this usually causes few problems and can usually be avoided by not wearing a belt as the pregnancy progresses. Occasionally, at the end of the third trimester, the ileostomy may be displaced from the enlarging uturus, resulting in a partial obstruction of the small intestine. This may require the induction of labor a little earlier than the expected date of delivery.

Summary

Women with IBD who have inactive disease or disease that is under good control with medication can look forward to an uncomplicated pregnancy and the delivery of a healthy, full-term baby. It is wise to plan the timing of pregnancy with your physician in order to achieve a remission before conception. If a flare-up of the disease occurs during pregnancy, you should not be reluctant to accept routine medical treatment. Taking most IBD medications during pregnancy will not pose a threat to the fetus; treatment may induce a remission of symptoms and will allow the pregnancy to continue with the best possible outcome.

Coping with IBD in the Later Years

13

If the challenges of IBD appear daunting to young people, imagine how they must seem to a person who is perhaps age 50 and at the peak of productivity, or age 60 or 70 and looking forward to enjoying the retirement years. Although both Crohn's disease and ulcerative colitis begin most often in adolescence or young adulthood, approximately 5 to 15 percent of people with IBD develop it later in life. As people live longer, however, and as the proportion of older people in our society grows, the number of people with late-onset IBD is also likely to grow.

Making the Correct Diagnosis

Part of the problem is deciding whether an older person coming to the physician with the usual signs of IBD—abdominal pain, diarrhea, rectal bleeding, fever—actually has IBD or some other bowel problem unrelated to IBD. As the bowel ages, it is prone to a number of disorders whose symptoms closely resemble those of ulcerative colitis or Crohn's disease. What are these disorders and how are they differentiated from IBD?

The most common of these is **infectious colitis,** an inflammation of the colon usually caused by bacteria. In order to exclude or "rule out" this form of colitis, the physician needs to obtain stool specimens to test for these bacteria, as well as their sensitivity to specific antibiotics. This test is called culture and sensitivity (C&S), and is discussed in

Chapter 2. Infectious colitis usually lasts no longer than two weeks, resolves by itself, or responds to antibiotic treatment. However, antibiotics themselves can cause colitis. This kind of colitis, **antibiotic-associated colitis,** can develop when the antibiotic unintentionally kills off certain helpful bacteria in the colon, thus permitting the overgrowth of **pathogenic** or disease-causing bacteria usually kept in check by the normal colonic bacteria. Infectious colitis is not a chronic condition and usually resolves after discontinuing the offending antibiotic or using other antibiotics, if necessary.

A condition called **ischemic colitis** occurs almost exclusively in older people and may resemble IBD very closely. The term "ischemia" means insufficient blood flow, and many people with ischemic colitis also have some form of cardiovascular disease. It is this prior condition that often leads to diminished blood flow to a portion of the colon.

The onset of ischemic colitis is usually quite sudden, with mild crampy pain in the left lower part of the abdomen, followed by bloody diarrhea. Distention (bloating) of the abdomen, vomiting, and constipation can also occur. The physician can usually make the diagnosis of ischemic colitis by taking a careful medical history and performing tests such as a colonoscopy and/or a barium enema. Most episodes of ischemic colitis resolve on their own and do not recur; some require surgery. If ischemic colitis becomes chronic, it can become quite difficult to tell it apart from IBD.

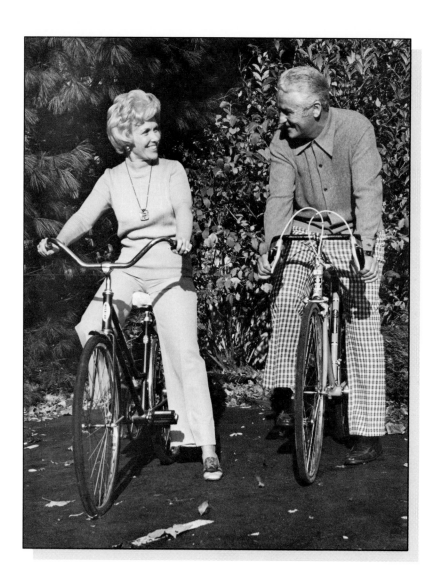

*Like Crohn's disease, diverticulitis
may cause abdominal pain,
fever, a mass that can be felt
in the abdomen, and fistulas.*

Diverticulosis, the presence of
numerous out-pouchings in the bowel wall,
is also very common among older people.
Diverticulosis causes no symptoms and
people are usually unaware of this condition
until the tiny pouches become inflamed,
resulting in **diverticulitis,** or cause
bleeding. Like Crohn's disease, diverticulitis
may cause abdominal pain, fever, a mass
that can be felt in the abdomen, and fistulas.
An attack of diverticulitis usually comes on
suddenly while Crohn's disease of the colon
usually has a slower onset. The bleeding
caused by diverticular disease is swift and
self-limited, although it may require surgery
to correct; in Crohn's colitis, bleeding is
frequent, sporadic, and mixed with diarrhea.

Two recently described forms of colitis
that may masquerade as IBD are
collagenous colitis and **microscopic
colitis.** Collgenous colitis causes a chronic,
watery diarrhea and may be accompanied
by abdominal pain, nausea, vomiting, and
weight loss. Most of the people diagnosed
with this rare disorder have been women
near age 60. Although the symptoms
resemble those of IBD, the colon looks
completely normal through the endoscope.
However, biopsies reveal a thicker than
normal layer of connective tissue (collagen)
just beneath the inner surface of bowel.
Microscopic colitis is very similar to
collagenous colitis, except for the absence
of the thickened collagen layer and the
presence of inflammatory cells. Some
experts believe that the two diseases are but
a spectrum of one disease.

Lastly, the prolonged use of anti-inflammatory drugs such as Advil,® Motrin,® and Naprosyn,® used by many mature adults to combat the aches and pains of arthritis, can produce lesions in the intestine that look just like those of Crohn's disease. Use of these medications can even bring about a relapse of pre-existing Crohn's disease that was previously in remission.

In trying to determine whether you have Crohn's disease or ulcerative colitis, your physician should take all these other potential diseases into consideration, a process known as **differential diagnosis.** Often, the presence of extra-intestinal symptoms, such as particular skin lesions or ulcers (erythema nodosum or pyoderma gangrenosum), eye problems (iritis), mouth sores (aphthous stomatitis), or non-deforming arthritis will help to confirm the physician's suspicion of IBD. If there is disease activity (fissures or fistulas) around the anal area, the most likely diagnosis is Crohn's disease.

In making the diagnosis, your physician uses the same tools and tests he/she would use in a younger person (See Chapter 2)—only more carefully. Sometimes, for example, a sigmoidoscopic examination can substitute for a full colonoscopy, which can be performed at a later date when symptoms have subsided. Since there are often other unrelated physical problems that accompany bowel symptoms, your physician will use great caution in performing any test that might be too strenuous or stressful for you.

Treating IBD in Older Adults

Just as the escalating medical problems associated with aging can make it difficult to arrive at a diagnosis of IBD, they can also complicate the treatment of IBD. The medications—sulfasalazine, 5-ASA, corticosteroids, immunosuppressives, etc.—are the same as those used to treat younger patients. However, some problems

of aging, such as diabetes, hypertension (high blood pressure), osteoporosis (thinning of the bones), and some forms of heart disease, can be made worse by taking steroids. Steroids tend to raise blood sugar, increase blood pressure through salt and water retention, and can further deplete calcium in the bones, leading to fractures. Immunosuppressive medications can be substituted for steroids or can allow their doses to be lowered gradually.

When an older person with IBD needs surgery, early operation is recommended.

When surgery is required to control symptoms, older people with IBD do as well as their younger counterparts. In fact, most surgeons prefer to operate sooner rather than later in older patients because it is easier for them to tolerate surgery than to suffer acute symptoms and prolonged use of medications. This is particularly true for ulcerative colitis, since onset of symptoms is often sudden and severe, and removal of the colon provides the only complete cure. In this case, the operation of choice is colectomy with standard ileostomy; few surgeons will perform an ileoanal anastomosis (pull-through operation) in a person over 50, mainly because muscle tone in the anal sphincter declines with age.

Likewise, when an older person with Crohn's disease needs surgery, early operation is recommended. This might be a resection with anastomosis (reconnection); more than likely, this surgery will involve the colon, since Crohn's colitis is even more common in older patients than it is in the young. If more extensive surgery, such as colectomy with ileostomy is needed, it can be done in stages to allow for fewer post-operative complications, a faster return to good nutritional status, and a speedy recovery.

What is the Outlook for the Older Person with IBD?

The outlook for the older person with IBD is good and getting better. Although there are some deaths as a result of the sudden onset of either ulcerative colitis or Crohn's disease, or because surgery is delayed too long, these are the exception rather than the rule. The increased awareness on the part of physicians that a new onset of IBD is possible in the later years has already improved the survival of older patients. Further improvements in longevity and quality of life surely will follow the development of new medical treatments and newer surgical techniques.

Part IV

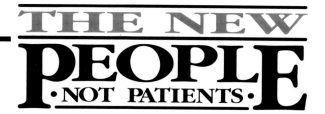

THE NEW
PEOPLE
·NOT PATIENTS·

Your Special Needs
as a Person with IBD

Communicating with Your Doctor

14

C rohn's disease and ulcerative colitis are serious chronic illnesses. Until the cause and cure are known, you can anticipate recurrences from time to time. When you "flare-up," often without notice, you can expect interruptions in your daily activities that may have a debilitating emotional and physical impact. Early on, it is crucial that you establish a relationship with an understanding physician, one capable of providing you with the best medical treatment and emotional support to help you obtain the best possible quality of life. The comfort level at which you interact with your doctor will have an important effect on the way you are able to deal with your illness.

The Value of Asking Questions

A recent study of people with chronic illnesses found that those who took a more active role in communicating with their physicians coped well with their disease on a daily basis. Those patients who became assertive in seeking information had a greater part in making the decisions that influenced their health and medical treatment. On the other hand, patients who remained relatively uninformed and did not take an active role in their care were less prepared to integrate treatment programs into workable daily routines and less able to cope with their illnesses.

It is a real challenge for the person with IBD to find a physician who has the medical approach and personality suited to a relationship that may last for many years.

Individuals' "need" levels vary, as do their personalities. You are the best one to assess your individual needs as you select a physician and structure your personal support system. Some patients deny illnesses, avoid office visits, and expect their physicians to do only what is minimally required to keep them well. Others require frequent reassurance on the telephone, numerous office visits, and a doctor who is available at all times to answer questions. Some people respond well to the physician who takes an intellectual, scholarly approach to treatment, while others need one with a more personal, caring approach. It is a real challenge for the person with IBD to find a physician who has the medical approach and personality suited to a relationship that may last for many years. Mutual trust is the major component in this relationship: for the patient, trust that the physician is competent and compassionate; for the physician, trust that the patient will be honest and forthright and will become a true partner in the treatment process. Finding the right physician to care for your IBD is a challenge worth pursuing.

What to Expect of Your Physician

You need to be able to talk to your doctor. Your physician should be accessible to you, either personally, through an associate, or through a member of the office staff. You should be able to contact the office during the day, at night, during weekends, and especially in case of an emergency. When you visit the office, you should expect knowledgeable treatment of your illness. He/she should be sensitive to your emotional and physical well-being and should be willing to talk frankly about the outlook for the future and the goals that you will set together . You can expect your physician to discuss the signs and symptoms of your illness you will feel. It is a good idea to ask your physician to provide a drawing of the areas of involvement of your bowel. You should expect your physician to discuss your medications, how long they will take to be effective, what are the side effects, and exactly what time of day they should be taken (See Chapter 5 for details about IBD medications).

In addition, you should expect your doctor to discuss your health related quality of life, which is the impact that any illness has on a single individual. In addition to finding out how you are doing, your physician should be prepared to discuss how IBD has affected your life in terms of social, sexual and physical functioning. It may also be important to discuss how the illness has affected those closest to you.

Who Should Be Your Physician

As a person with IBD, it is in your best interest to try to identify a board-certified gastroenterologist (or pediatric gastroenterologist) in your community, and if possible, one who has a specific interest in inflammatory bowel disease. This information is available to you through the local, regional or national office of the Crohn's and Colitis Foundation of America (CCFA), which maintains a current physician roster of more than 1500 qualified physicians interested in IBD. Being board-certified means that your physician has spent the required number of years in a recognized and approved training program in internal medicine and gastroenterology (usually four to five years) and has passed examinations given by both the boards of internal medicine and gastroenterology. You can also call the state or county medical society and ask for the names of qualified physicians who have special training or who have indicated a strong interest in the management of inflammatory bowel disease. Each public library has a directory of licensed physicians listed by specialty.

If your city or town does not have a gastroenterologist, a second good choice is an internist or family practice physician who is experienced in treating patients with IBD. Many physicians who are not board-certified in gastroenterology can manage IBD problems. If and when difficulties arise in treatment, these physicians can then obtain advice from consulting gastroenterologists or surgeons who specialize in treating IBD.

Most physicians display their diplomas in their office. If they are not readily visible, you have the right to ask your physician where he/she attended medical school, completed medical internship and residency, and whether he or she is board-certified in gastroenterology.

The Office Visit

Every physician's office should have a comfortable, well ventilated waiting room, clean, private examining rooms, and accessible bathrooms. The office staff should be courteous, sensitive and understanding. When discussing medical or financial matters, they should talk quietly to ensure privacy. They should address you in a way that makes you feel comfortable, and if you have strong feelings about the way you are addressed by the physician or staff, you have every right to say so. Some patients prefer to be addressed more formally while others prefer the use of first names. Your preference should be made clear to the physicians and the staff. If you note a recurring problem in the way the office is managed, it is appropriate to tell your physician about this, either in person or with a short note.

Your physician should be on time for an appointment. This is often difficult, since no physician refuses an urgent telephone call from a patient, from a colleague requiring immediate advice, or from a nurse reporting a change in the condition of a hospitalized patient. If you are the person who is waiting, try to understand the possible reasons for the interruptions. At another time, it could be you. However, if the physician is delayed, it is not inappropriate for you to inquire how long it will take to be seen and whether the appointment should be rescheduled.

After being examined, you should have the opportunity to discuss your care with the physician in the consultation room with the door closed and without telephone interruptions. This may not take place after every visit, but the opportunity should be available when there are important issues to discuss or decisions to be made. It is preferable to have a family member or friend sit in the consultation with you at these important times. Physicians prefer to have a third party present in order to help the patient review objectively what was discussed.

Your physician should have a supply of literature available for you to read to learn more about your illness. The CCFA provides its physician members with brochures, books, videotapes and slides to help to bring you up to date on the manifestations, complications and therapy of your illness.

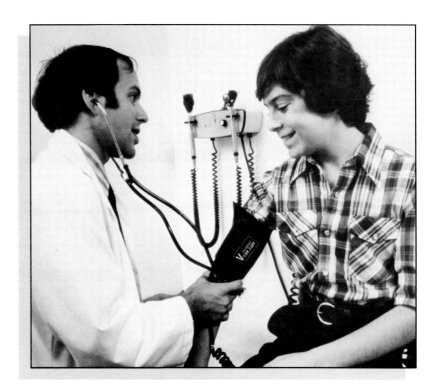

What Your Physician Expects of You

In a partnership of mutual trust, you should not expect an immediate response from your physician for a routine problem. You should understand that physicians are frequently busy and must take care of emergency problems first, urgent cases second, and routine problems last. If you need an immediate response, you should state this clearly to the physician's representative, whether it is his/her office staff or the answering service. If a response is not needed until the end of the day or until the next day, you should make that clear as well. Inform the office or the answering service of the best time for the physician to return your call and try and make sure that no one is using the phone at that time. *Telephone calls on weekends and evenings are for urgent and emergency problems only.* In these situations you may reach an associate of the physician who is "on call" and may not know the specific details of your medical problem. Therefore, if the problem can wait until the next day, you may be better off waiting and talking to your own physician.

Most physicians feel that patients should know the details of the medications they are taking, including the names, dosages and the times they are to be taken.

You should request renewals of your medications with adequate time for the physician to respond. If renewal of a medication is complex, it is a good idea to send a note to the physician outlining the requirements. This is especially important if you are planning to be away for a prolonged time. Most physicians feel that patients should know the details of the medications they are taking, including the names, dosages and the times they are to be taken. If you have trouble remembering, keep a list in your purse or wallet detailing your use of medication.

Whether you are telephoning your physician or visiting the office, you should have a very clear, concise, and pertinent list of questions to ask. Very long lists are not appropriate. Physicians are people, too, and may become weary or impatient when faced with exhausting questions at each visit or phone call. Decide what is important before contacting your physician and try and keep phone call time to a minimum.

You should also tell your physician which person should be kept informed about your progress. This can be a parent, spouse or close friend, or any other person you wish. A physician will not respond to requests for information from a family member unless you have given prior permission for him/her to disclose this information. As noted above, it is advisable for this family member or friend to accompany you on medical visits, since he or she can work with you and your physician in reaching important decisions about diagnostic procedures, a significant change in therapy, hospitalization, or surgery.

While you are in your doctor's office, you may notice that the staff is often overworked and may be dealing with urgent situations. Nurses and secretaries may conceal the fact that there are serious problems that have them very worried. If the office staff appears to be under pressure, hold your routine concerns until a later time. Taking the time to get to know and respect the office staff can be of great help when you are trying to reach your doctor.

Finally, remember, the physician is a person too. Just like you, he or she has family and social obligations, outside interests, good days and not so good days. Your respect and sensitivity for his/her personal life and privacy will be appreciated and returned.

Improving Your Health-Related Quality of Life

Your health related quality of life is the impact IBD will have on you as an individual. There are several ways to improve your health-related quality of life and your physician will expect you to be a partner in this process. To assure yourself of the best results of your treatment, comply with the prescribed medications and keep your physician informed of any side effects that may be affecting your well-being or your ability to continue on the medication.

Keep well-informed about your disease. Being familiar with the illness and what to expect of it in the future will tend to reduce your worries and concerns and will help you adjust to IBD. Take responsibility for your health care. For example, most treatment decisions involve choices: which medication to use, when to consider surgery, and even when to have tests performed. If your physician suggests that you undergo a particular test, he would expect you to ask the following question: "What do you expect to learn from this test that will alter the manner in which you are treating my case?" Tests can be time consuming, expensive and sometimes not so pleasant. You should play a role in deciding when these tests will be performed.

If you feel emotionally distressed, it is important to discuss this with your doctor. For example, emotional states like anxiety or depression lower your tolerance to pain. Counseling by your physician or referral to a therapist or support group will not only relieve your feelings of distress but may also improve your ability to cope with symptoms.

Choosing a Surgeon

When necessary, your primary physician will call on a surgeon for a consultation about your treatment. Personality and compatibility are important qualities in a surgeon, but they are not nearly as important as his/her surgical skill. The surgeon of your choice should be someone with a combination of experience and common sense. You should ask about important details, such as the surgeon's academic credentials, experience in performing surgery in IBD, and the number of similar operations he or she has performed in the preceding year. You should not be afraid to ask these questions; they are not impolite and are crucial in deciding whether to use this particular surgeon.

Personality and compatibility are important qualities in a surgeon, but they are not nearly as important as surgical skill.

There are also many questions you need to ask about the surgery itself. First, you should ask who will be actually performing the surgery: this surgeon, an associate or a surgical resident? At some large teaching institutions, physicians delegate some of the surgical procedures to senior resident surgeons in training. These surgeons may have four to five or more years of experience and are highly qualified. You should also ask who will be giving you your postoperative care, both in the hospital and after discharge. This is particularly important if one of the newer surgical alternatives, such as an ileoanal anastomosis or continent ileostomy, is being considered. In most major hospitals where these alternatives are performed, enterostomal therapists (E.T.s) are available for your consultation and work closely with the physician in your postoperative care.

When a decision to operate has been reached, the surgeon should discuss the "major" potential complications of the surgery well before of the date of your operation. If the surgeon does not initiate this discussion, you should feel free to ask any of the questions you need answered. Minor complications occur frequently after surgery and you should not expect your surgeon to discuss every possible thing that can occur; most surgeons limit themselves to the major potential complications of an operation. Before surgery, you will be asked to sign a consent form, a medical-legal document certifying that you understand the nature of the operation and its possible complications. Make sure that you are well-informed and really do understand the procedure that is about to be performed.

Finally, you should be told the cost of the procedure and follow-up care. If there are questions about your insurance coverage, these should be discussed *before* the surgery with your surgeon or the office staff. Any requests for a reduced fee, for whatever reason, should be made in advance.

When to Get a Consultation

Even in the best patient-doctor relationship, there may be a need for a second opinion with a gastroenterologist or surgeon. There are many valid reasons for this second opinion. For example, there may be rapid deterioration in the pattern of your illness, or your condition may not be responding to current medical treatment. You may not be extremely ill but you may be looking for newer alternative management to improve your quality of life. As a result, your physician may be ready to suggest a major change in the course of your therapy, such as the introduction of a new medication, hyperalimentation, hospitalization, or even surgery.

It is far better to discuss the request for a second opinion with your physician than to obtain a consultation without his or her knowledge.

During the past few years, there has been a much-needed surge of newer treatments for IBD. These include new drugs, including several 5-ASA compounds (administered both orally and rectally), and a new generation of immunosuppressives (See Chapter 5). Also, newer surgical alternative techniques have been developed for both ulcerative colitis and Crohn's disease. Since less is known about the long-term effects of these medications and surgical techniques, your physician may be the one to suggest a consultation with a gastroenterologist or surgeon who has been more actively involved in bringing these advances to the public. Although your physician will often suggest this consultation, a good doctor should never feel hurt or threatened if *you* request the consultation. Such a request may even increase the sense of shared responsibility between doctor and patient. It is far better to discuss the request for a second opinion with your physician than to obtain a consultation without his or her knowledge. Should this occur, your physician may sense a lack of trust which will influence your relationship from that point on.

Regardless of who initiates the request for consultation, your physician should give you the name of several reliable physicians to consult. Your physician should then make your records and x-rays available and ideally make the initial telephone call to familiarize the consultant with your case. Whenever possible, you should hand carry as much information to the consultant as you are able. This includes a copy of a referral letter, your records, your x-ray folder and operative reports. Having the information sent may result in delays or loss of this important material in the mail. Since you are the legal "owner" of the information contained in your office records and x-rays, you will need to sign a release form to legalize the transfer of this information.

When seeing a consultant, be prepared to present your medical history, including the time of onset, pattern of illness, dates of admissions to hospitals, surgical procedures, types of medications and dosages. If possible, this information should be given in chronological order. It may be helpful to bring a concise written history containing this information in outline form. Be clear, logical and specific about why you are seeking the consultation. It is important to bring a family member or close friend to this consultation. This person will often be able to help you with the details and hear more objectively what the consultant is telling you. This will allow you to discuss the recommendations and avoid misinterpretation after you have left the doctor's office.

Following the history, you should receive a full physical examination and should have enough time in the consultation room to answer all your questions. After the visit, the consulting physician will write a letter to your physician summarizing his/her findings and recommendations. You are entitled to a copy of this consultation letter. You should then call or see your physician to discuss the recommendations. If the consultant has agreed with the plans initially outlined by your physician, you and your physician should be reassured. If there are differences, further discussion and additional input from yet another physician may be required to chart the appropriate course for your therapy.

Sometimes, even under the best of circumstances, you may become dissatisfied with the care you are receiving from your physician. If this happens, you have every right to find another physician whose approach may be better suited to your needs. In this situation, you should inform your treating physician that you are seeking help elsewhere and ask him/her to provide a summary of your case as well as copies of all pertinent medical information. Inflammatory bowel disease is a frustrating illness for both patient and physician and a change in physician may at times be helpful.

Good Medical Care When You Can't Afford It

If your medical insurance has lapsed at the time of a flare-up or if you have no coverage for office visits, consider visiting the gastroenterology clinic at a major medical center. As a general rule, these clinics are staffed by gastrointestinal residents under the supervision of a senior gastroenterologist. The chances are that you will be seen by a physician who is already qualified in internal medicine and is working toward certification in gastroenterology. Your x-rays will often be performed by a radiology resident supervised by an attending radiologist and such procedures as upper gastrointestinal endoscopy, sigmoidoscopy and colonoscopy will once again be performed under the supervision of an experienced senior physician. A clinic physician will take a history and perform a physical examination and you will be followed regularly at fees decided according to your ability to pay. There are also a few private clinics that are willing to perform a similar service. The CCFA can provide you with a list of clinics in your geographical area.

Some private physicians treat patients at reduced rates. If the doctor agrees, be honest about the limitations of your financial resources. Make a concerted effort to pay something every month, even if it is a small amount, to let the physician know that you have appreciated this courtesy to you. You might even consider volunteering to be part of IBD research projects conducted at major teaching institutions, including the testing of newer medications. At these centers, all research projects are scrutinized carefully by a research committee made up of physicians and lay people. These committees are set up to see that no harm is done to patients who are participating in research projects, and you will be carefully monitored under guidelines of the federal Privacy Act. If you are a good candidate for a particular project, you will be assured of good follow-up care on a regular basis by qualified physicians.

Danger Signals: When to Call Your Doctor

It is useful to separate telephone calls to your physician into three categories: routine, urgent and emergency. Your doctor should always inform you of the best time to place routine calls to the office. Routine calls are made to obtain the results of blood and laboratory tests or to report any changes in symptoms or a response to medication. Your doctor will want to note the nature of your call on your chart so it is important to call at a time when he or she is in the office and the chart is available.

When you call your physician's office with an urgent call, be prepared to be as specific as possible with the office staff.

An urgent call is one that is important but is not a true emergency. This kind of call should be returned by your doctor on the same day. An example of a reason for an urgent call might be the sudden appearance of a rash on your body. This rash might indicate an allergic reaction to a medication or even a new symptom of the illness itself, such as erythema nodosum (painful, tender bumps usually on your shins, indicating a flaring of the illness). Other urgent symptoms include swelling of the joints, persistent low grade fever, or the appearance of a small amount of blood in your stool. When you call your physician's office with an urgent call, be prepared to be as specific as possible with the office staff. Note that it is an urgent call, refrain from asking multiple questions, and stick to the nature of the urgency. You have the right to ask when you can expect a return call from your physician and be sure to stay off the telephone during these times.

An emergency phone call is justified by an acute, dramatic change in your illness. These changes include:

- a sudden high fever which might be accompanied by shaking chills
- a sudden weight loss of over five pounds in a few days
- the onset of significant or new rectal bleeding
- any severe abdominal pain that persists for longer than an hour
- persistent vomiting accompanied by cessation of bowel movements
- a drastic change in bowel movements without passing gas

It is essential that you convey the emergent nature of your call to the office staff. Your doctor should speak to you at once if he/she is there, or by return phone call.

If you are the type of person who can effectively determine the routine, urgent or emergency nature of your call, you will greatly enhance your relationship with your doctor and the office staff.

How to Eat
When You Have IBD

15

The importance of nutrition in maintaining or returning you to good health is a well-recognized concept of our time. Meeting nutritional needs is necessary for everyone, but is especially important for people with inflammatory bowel disease. There are several reasons why this is so. Medications are often more effective when your nutritional state is not depleted. In addition, when intestinal losses of proteins and other nutrients occur in IBD, they must be compensated for by increasing the amount of food taken in. The slowing of growth which occurs in some children and teenagers with IBD often responds dramatically to increases in the intake of protein and calories. Weight loss in IBD can also affect the body's hormones: in women and girls, this can result in irregular periods or the temporary cessation of the menstrual cycle. Being able to eat sufficient quantities of food is often very difficult when gastrointestinal symptoms are active. In this chapter, we will present several approaches that have been helpful in maximizing food intake in IBD.

Being able to eat sufficient quantities of food is often very difficult when gastrointestinal symptoms are active.

Facts and Fallacies about Nutrition in IBD

Nutitional requirements for an individual with IBD will vary with age, sex, physical activity level and any excessive losses caused by intestinal inflammation and diarrhea. The first step in individual counseling is for a dietitian or nutritionist to analyze your nutrient intake. This is usually accomplished by completing a "food diary" over a period of days or weeks. If you are eating less than the recommended amount for a healthy person of your age, size, etc., (based upon Recommended Daily Allowances or RDA), then you will need to find ways to increase your intake of food.

If you are having trouble gaining or maintaining your weight, you may need even more calories than the RDAs require. It is important to recognize that the amounts of some nutrients (calories, protein, vitamins and minerals) that are needed by the body increase from childhood through adolescence and then decrease during adulthood. Recommendations for nutrient intake must be increased further if there is evidence of excessive losses of fat, protein, iron, calcium, or zinc, or if chronic undernutrition has resulted in depleted body stores of these nutrients. The recommended amounts of calories and protein for healthy individuals appear in the following chart.

Usually, the nutritional needs of the person with IBD can be met by food alone, together with a well-formulated multivitamin

Recommended Dietary Allowances

		Average Daily Caloric Intake (kilocalories)	Average Daily Protein Intake (grams)
Children	(7–10 yrs)	2000	28
Males	(11–14 yrs)	2500	45
	(15–18 yrs)	3000	59
	(19–24 yrs)	2900	58
	(25–50 yrs)	2900	63
	(51–75 yrs)	2300	63
Females	(11–14 yrs)	2200	46
	(15–18 yrs)	2200	44
	(19–24 yrs)	2200	46
	(25–50 yrs)	2200	50
	(51–75 yrs)	1900	50

Source: Food and Nutrition Board, National Academy of Sciences National Research Council, Revised 1989.

and, if needed, additional supplemental iron. It is important to recognize that it is the *total daily intake* of calories, protein and other nutrients, not the amount eaten at mealtimes, that determines whether you are eating enough. Therefore, if you feel full at mealtimes, frequent smaller meals with snacks may meet your nutritional needs.

Parents sometimes consider the "fast foods" enjoyed by their children or teenagers unhealthy "junk foods." However, some of these foods have substantial nutritional value. A slice of pizza provides protein, calcium and vitamin D from the cheese, vitamins A and C from the tomato sauce, and B vitamins from the crust. Similarly, hamburgers and cheeseburgers provide plenty of protein in addition to calories. While these foods contain more fat and salt than is wise on a long-term basis, the calories and protein they provide during the growing period can help to maintain normal gains in height and weight for young people with IBD.

Milk products like cheese, milk shakes and ice cream are excellent sources of calcium, calories and protein and should not be avoided simply because a child or adult has IBD. In people with low intestinal levels of the enzyme lactase, milk sugar (lactose) may cause bloating or diarrhea (lactose intolerance). Discomfort is temporary, however, and can usually be alleviated with the use of a commercially prepared enzyme (See below). There is no evidence to suggest that these products will aggravate IBD.

Some people with IBD limit their intake of food during daytime hours in order to prevent cramping, trips to the bathroom, or accidents at work or school. Unfortunately, this practice can greatly reduce the number of calories consumed each day. If the physician is made aware of this situation, specific medications can be prescribed and arrangements made with teachers or employers. The CCFA pamphlet for teachers is very helpful in explaining the special needs of children with IBD while they are at school.

At times, the symptoms of IBD can prevent you from eating enough to satisfy nutritional requirements. This can happen when there is a narrowing of the bowel or continuous diarrhea. Eating is often difficult under these circumstances, so liquid formula supplements may be used to provide additional nutrients. Many products are now available in a range of flavors and prices. Your doctor may prescribe an elemental formula when a more digested protein or lower residue diet is necessary. Chapter 16 contains a complete list of these products.

How to Decrease Intestinal Cramping Associated with Eating

When IBD is active, it is not unusual for eating to cause cramping and intestinal discomfort. This is especially true when the small intestine is inflamed. Since there are several reasons why this occurs (as described below), it is important to observe any association between specific foods or types of foods and the onset of gastrointestinal symptoms. Any of the following foods can cause discomfort:

Milk and milk products. Lactase is an enzyme in the small intestine which breaks down lactose, the sugar found in dairy products. If lactase levels are low, symptoms of bloating, gas and/or diarrhea usually occur 30 to 90 minutes after drinking milk or eating large amounts of cheese or ice cream. Some dairy products with small amounts of lactose, like butter, yogurt and hard cheeses (swiss, muenster, cheddar) cause few problems. Using non-dairy (milk substitute) products, taking commercially available lactase in capsules, or adding it to

What Happens during Digestion

As food is eaten, it undergoes both *physical* and *chemical* breakdown by the digestive organs. Digestion begins in the mouth as chewing breaks up large food particles and saliva transforms starch into glucose or simple sugar. The esophagus is a muscular tube which propels the food to the stomach in wave-like movements called **peristalsis.** There it is rhythmically churned and further broken down physically by acid secretions. Interestingly, stomach acid also kills most of the harmful bacteria that may have been swallowed with the food. The stomach also secretes **pepsin,** a powerful enzyme which begins the complex breakdown of proteins.

From the stomach, food enters the upper part of the small intestine, the **duodenum,** where it encounters bile from the liver and enzymes from the pancreas which enter the lumen and continue the digestive process. These secretions further reduce the complex proteins, fats and carbohydrates we eat, turning them into **amino acids, fatty acids** and **simple sugars,** which can be readily absorbed and used by the body.

The **jejunum,** or mid-small intestine, is the site of absorption of most of the intestinal contents. Although a normal small intestine ranges from 12 to about 20 feet in length, the absorptive surface area is greatly increased because of the finger-like projections, called **villi,** which line the inner surface of the lumen. Absorption continues in the lower small intestine, or **ileum,** where vitamins A, D, E, K, and B_{12} are also absorbed.

When entering the **cecum,** or first part of the colon, intestinal contents are quite liquid. The colon then acts to reabsorb water and salt into the body and to propel the now solid waste material towards the **rectum** where it signals the urge to defecate.

milk for 24 to 48 hours before drinking, will help alleviate these symptoms. Recently, enzymatically-treated (predigested) milk and non-dairy frozen desserts have become available in grocery stores.

High fiber foods. This category includes foods such as seeds, nuts, popcorn, corn, and certain Chinese vegetables. These foods may produce cramping if there is narrowing of the bowel. When this occurs early in the course of the disease, it is often a temporary problem caused by edema or swelling of the bowel wall. Later in the course of the illness, these symptoms may indicate scarring (stenosis) of the intestine. High fiber foods also contribute to diarrhea (greater stool volume) because they are incompletely digested by the small intestine. Once fiber enters the large intestine, it stimulates contractions, especially when the colon is inflamed with either Crohn's colitis or ulcerative colitis. This is the reason for using "low residue" foods such as broth, gelatin, poultry without skin, potatoes without skin, rolls, noodles, rice, eggs and fish. High fiber foods may also contribute to diarrhea by causing mechanical irritation if the colon is severely inflamed. A more complete discussion of this topic can be found in the following chapter.

Fried or greasy foods. This category includes pork products, butter, margarine, cream sauces etc. These foods may cause gas and diarrhea if fat absorption is incomplete. Usually this occurs after removal of large amounts of small bowel, especially ileum. One way to overcome these symptoms is to decrease the amount of fat in the diet. Another way is to use an easily absorbable fat, such as medium-chain triglyceride (MCT) oil, in cooking and salad dressings.

Large meals. Many people with IBD find that frequent (perhaps five) small meals produce fewer symptoms than the customary three large meals per day. From a nutritional point of view, what matters most is the total number of calories, protein and calcium consumed daily. Despite attention to all of these factors, intestinal discomfort may continue to recur with eating. If this happens, an adjustment in medication may help alleviate the symptoms. Corticosteroid medications such as prednisone may significantly decrease intestinal inflammation and allow the bowel to function more normally. Other medications (such as antispasmodics and antidiarrheal medications) decrease cramping and stool liquidity and frequency. When taken 15 to 20 minutes before eating, these medications decrease symptoms that interrupt meals, thus encouraging greater intake of food. They are most helpful in mild disease but must be used with caution, if at all, in severely active disease because of the possibility of causing excessive dilatation of the bowel (megacolon).

Sometimes, despite repeated attempts at eating, nutritional status deteriorates in IBD. Weight loss may persist and body stores of muscle, fat and protein diminish. In children and teenagers, the growth rate may slow to below normal. Faced with problems such as these, the physician may adjust the medication schedule or reconsider the option of surgery.

Other Ways to Increase Nutritional Intake

In some circumstances, nutritional support can be enhanced by alternative means. One method involves the infusion of liquid formulas directly into the stomach or small bowel through a small, soft feeding tube. Usually the tube is inserted into the nostril and passed into the stomach each night. It is removed in the morning so that the person can go to school or work. If hospitalization is required, the infusion may continue on a 24-hour basis. This approach has been used successfully to control inflammation and to improve growth in children either alone or in combination with food intake during the day. As an alternative, some physicians have used nighttime gastrostomy feedings. A gastrostomy is a surgically-made opening through the abdominal wall directly into the stomach, through which the feeding tube is passed. The obvious advantage of this type of feeding is that it is not necessary to pass a tube through the nose each night.

When tube feeding is required, the composition of the liquid formula and the amount infused depend upon the needs of the individual. Short-term results (four to six weeks) with nasogastric infusion are usually good, indicating improvement in disease activity and growth. Understandably, the acceptance of tube feeding varies and may be higher in children than in adolescents and adults. However, adolescents may be highly motivated to comply with this regimen once they see consistent increases in weight and height, especially if plotted on standard growth curves.

A second method of supplying nutrient requirements is by vein (intravenous route). This approach bypasses the intestine altogether and "rests" the bowel by decreasing the work of digestion and intestinal blood flow. This method has been called intravenous "hyperalimentation" in the past, but is now called total parenteral nutrition (TPN).

TPN can be used temporarily in the hospital or adapted for on-going use at home. Usually the intravenous administration continues during the night but is stopped in the morning so that the person can go to school or work. TPN is expensive, requires a training program in the hospital, and is therefore recommended only in selected situations, such as preparing malnourished patients for surgery, healing severe perianal inflammation or fistulous disease, or reversing growth failure unresponsive to oral nutrition. The

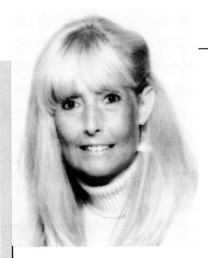

Audrey Kron

Medical psychotherapist and marriage counselor Audrey Kron manages to lead a full and rewarding life despite being on home total parenteral nutrition (TPN). She is "on the pump" for 18 hours one night a week, 14 hours two nights a week, and for 10 hours on three other nights, but she doesn't let it stop her from working, travelling, volunteering, and enjoying a full social life. Although she found being on TPN "overwhelming" at first, Audrey says, "As I became more experienced, it has become part of my daily routine. I'm now even more determined to enjoy myself, and thankful for the good times." As with most things in life, she adds, "It's what you can do that's important, not what you can't do."

technique should be supervised only by a medical team familiar with its management. Currently, this requires a group effort consisting of physician, nurse, nutritionist and pharmacist.

Many approaches are available to maintain or improve the nutritional status of the person with IBD. The easiest and safest methods should be used first whenever possible, with the more invasive approaches reserved for special circumstances. Your continual good nutrition depends upon maintaining communication with your gastroenterologist and with a nutritionist or dietitian.

A Guide to Food Sources of Essential Nutrients

16

Nutrition is an environmental factor which continually affects health and disease. It is important to remember that as far as we know, no food causes IBD, and that dietary modification can actually help reduce disease symptoms and replace lost nutrients. Once IBD is in remission, eating habits can often return to normal. While the health team that cares for you will be the best guide to developing your specific dietary plan, we present the following information to help you choose foods and supplements to carry out that plan.

It is important to remember that as far as we know, no food causes IBD, and that dietary modification can actually help reduce disease symptoms and replace lost nutrients.

Basic Nutritional Requirements

The body makes thousands of different substances daily, but the "essential nutrients" it cannot produce must be provided by the food we eat. These nutrients are made from 25 chemical elements, 11 of which—carbon, hydrogen, oxygen, nitrogen, phosphorus, calcium, sulfur, sodium, potassium, magnesium and chloride—make up 99 percent of the human body. These elements are the building blocks of proteins, fats, carbohydrates, vitamins, water and nucleic acids. They form our bones and teeth and are essential parts of all cells and body fluids. The remaining 1 percent of the body consists of the trace elements (copper, zinc, manganese, etc.) which are required in only tiny amounts, but are no less essential.

Nutritional requirements for the general population have been established by the Food and Nutrition Board of the National Research Council. They are called the Recommended Dietary Allowances (RDAs) and are the "levels of intake of essential nutrients considered to be adequate to meet the known nutritional needs of practically all healthy persons."

RDAs can be met by eating a specified number of servings from each of the Basic Four Food Groups:

- Meat and meat substitutes—2 servings
- Dairy—2–4 servings
- Cereal and grains—4 servings
- Fruits and vegetables—5 servings

Although RDAs are not specified for a particular individual or disease, they are useful as a starting point in planning nutritional programs for people with IBD. Modifications in diet are often required to lessen the symptoms of IBD, to meet the RDAs for specific nutrients, and to exceed the RDAs when it is necessary to correct nutritional deficiencies.

I. Dietary Modification in IBD

Nutritional deficiency in IBD may occur for the following reasons:

- Decreased food intake caused by symptoms or side effects of medications such as sulfasalazine or supplemental iron.

- Decreased absorption of food from the small intestine caused by inflammation or as a side effect of medications.
- Increased losses of protein or other substances that leak into the bowel lumen from diseased areas.

It is particularly important to be aware of drug-nutrient interactions. Sulfasalazine interferes with the absorption of folic acid, a water-soluble vitamin. High-dose daily corticosteroids can decrease intestinal absorption of calcium and phosphorus, increase urinary losses of vitamin C, calcium, potassium, zinc, and nitrogen, and cause excessive breakdown of protein. Steroids also cause fluid retention, an effect that can be counteracted by eating a diet lower in salt. A third important medication that may affect nutrients is cholestyramine (Questran®), which is sometimes helpful in controlling diarrhea caused by the presence of unabsorbed bile salts in the colon. (Bile salts are normally absorbed in the healthy ileum and recycled by the body.) Unfortunately, cholestyramine may also cause poor absorption of the fat soluble vitamins (A,D,E, and K) as well as folic acid, vitamin B-12, calcium, and iron. Awareness of these drug-nutrient interactions and increased intake of the nutrients affected can help prevent deficiencies.

The diets described below may be encountered at one time or another during the course of your treatment for IBD.

The Clear Liquid Diet

The clear liquid diet is helpful during intense disease activity, in transition between intravenous feeding and solid food, following surgery, or in preparation for diagnostic tests. This diet is highly restrictive but provides some calories, prevents dehydration, and reduces intestinal activity.

Foods Allowed:
- Boullion, fat-free broth
- Decaffeinated coffee
- Decaffeinated tea, herb teas
- Clear fruit juices and drinks (may need to be diluted with water to prevent diarrhea)
- Flavored or plain sparkling and mineral waters (may be mixed with juices to enhance flavor)
- Kool-aid (can be used to flavor commercial formulas)
- Popsicles (more nutritious when made from fruit juice or drinks)
- Gelatin (commercial products or homemade with clear juices)
- Carbonated beverages (without caffeine and allowed to flatten slightly)
- Honey, sugar, salt and flavorings

In addition, there are commercial semi-synthetic diets which may be allowed on your clear liquid diet. The palatability of these products is generally poor, but creative use of flavorings can significantly improve their acceptability. A word of caution: if you use these formulas on your clear liquid diet, be sure to drink them slowly, since they are concentrated and may cause cramping or diarrhea. Always check with your doctor before using these formulas.

Examples are:

Citrotein®
Criticare HN®
Pepti-2000®
Peptamen®
Precision Isotonic®
Precision Low Residue®
Reabilan, Reabilan HN®
Tolerex® (formerly Vivonex)®
Travasorb STD,® Travasorb HN®
Vital HN®
Vivonex T.E.N.® (Total Enteral Nutrition)

The Full Liquid Diet

The full liquid diet is traditionally used as a transition from clear liquid to solid food. This diet is more nutritious and palatable, and includes a greater variety of foods.

Foods Allowed:
Those on the Clear Liquid Diet plus:

- Milk, milk drinks, milk substitutes
- Cream and cream substitutes
- Eggs and egg substitutes used in custards, eggnogs, puddings.
- Fruit nectars
- Refined cooked cereals and strained whole grain cereals
- Puddings, ice cream, sherbet
- Vegetable juices
- Strained bland creamed meat, poultry and vegetable soups

The full liquid diet can be implemented entirely using commercially available formulas instead of the foods listed, or they can be used as supplements to increase the caloric and nutrient content of the diet.

A partial list of these products which can be taken orally includes:

Lactose-containing:

Carnation Instant Breakfast®
Complete Regular®
Meritene® Liquid & Powder
Nutrament®
Sustacal® Powder
Ensure® Pudding
Sustacal® Pudding

Lactose-free:
Ensure,® Ensure Plus,® Ensure Plus HN®
Isotein HN®
Sustacal® liquid, Sustacal HC®
   (high calorie)

What Is Enteral Nutrition?

Your physician may recommend a trial of enteral nutrition to decrease disease symptoms and improve your nutritional status if other dietary efforts have been unsuccessful. Enteral nutrition inolves using special liquid formulas for all or part of a day's dietary intake. They can be taken by mouth or sometimes through a soft nasogastric tube which is passed each night prior to nocturnal infusion during sleep. Studies have found this diet can reduce disease activity, allow lowering of medications, and improve nutritional status. This method has been most exciting in growth impaired children and adolescents. It allows full activity and regular mealtime during the day while providing those additional nutrients during the night that will promote growth and maturation. Formulas that have been used successfully include: Ensure,® Sustacal,® Osmolite HN,® Vivonex T.E.N.,® Vital HN.®

Additional products which are bland and unflavored, but can be used in preparing soups or flavored for drinking include:

Isocal,® Isocal HN® and Isocal HCN®
Osmolite,® Osmolite HN®
Magacal®
Travasorb,® Travasorb MCT®

The Lactose-Free Diet

Some individuals experience cramping, bloating and diarrhea when they consume milk because they are unable to adequately digest milk sugar (lactose). The full liquid diet is based on milk and milk products, so this poses a problem, but not an impossible one.

The intolerance to milk is caused by a deficiency of an intestinal enzyme called **lactase** which breaks down milk sugar (lactose) into two simple sugars that can be absorbed by the body. Those with diffuse small bowel disease may temporarily lack the enzyme, but in most cases an inherited trait causes loss of the enzyme with age, beginning usually around early adolescence. While some people cannot consume even small amounts of milk, in most people it is a dose-related phenomenon. Milk on cereal or ice cream may be fine, yet a whole glass of milk may produce symptoms. Yogurt is usually well-tolerated while buttermilk and acidophilus milk are not, even though they are cultured products as well.

Most symptoms can be prevented when lactase enzyme caplets (eg. Lactaid,® Dairy-Ease®) are taken simultaneously with foods that contain lactose, or when milk that has been pre-treated with commercially available lactase drops is used for drinking and in cooking.

Lactose-Free Foods:
Meat and Meat Substitute Group:

Eggs
Plain meats of all kinds
Poultry of all kinds
Fish of all kinds (fresh or canned)
Kosher hot dogs
Cold cuts

Fruit and vegetable group:

All plain fruits and vegetables (fresh, frozen or canned).

Bread and Cereal Group:

Breads, rolls, pastries (Some contain small amounts of milk or milk solids, but are rarely troublesome)
Cereal
Crackers
Pasta (macaroni, spaghetti, noodles)
Pretzels (Read ingredient labels carefully)

Dairy Group:

Butter*
Margarine*
(*May contain small amounts of milk, but are rarely troublesome.)
Non-dairy creamers (Note: Do not contain nutrients of milk—are only fat substitutes)
Soy milk and other soy dairy products

Soy milk is becoming available commercially and tofu can be used as a meat substitute or in place of cream cheese or sour cream in many products. There are delicious soy frozen desserts, such as Tofutti,® cheeses, and a yogurt-like product called Stir-Easy.®

Fats

   Salad dressings made without milk or
      milk products
   Vegetable oils
   Shortening
   Nut butters

Dairy Products with Minimal
Lactose Content:

Lactaid® treated milk: Lactaid,® a
commercially available lactase enzyme
predigests the lactose in milk before use.
The milk tastes slightly sweeter because
lactose is broken into two simpler,
sweeter-tasting sugars during digestion.

   Milk can be treated at home using
Lactaid® drops or purchased pre-treated in
your supermarket dairy case under the
Lactaid® trademark. The company also
makes cottage cheese and ice cream.

- *Margarine and Butter:* Contain trace
  amounts of lactose.
- *Cheese:* Blue, Brick, Camembert,
  Cheddar, Colby, Edam, Provolone,
  Swiss, pasteurized process American
  cheese all have "non-detectable"
  amounts of lactose. Cream cheese,
  cottage cheese and mozzarella contain
  small amounts of lactose but should
  not produce symptoms.
- *Ice Cream:* The very "richest" kinds
  have the least lactose, since they
  contain more cream than milk.

The Bland Diet

The bland diet is defined as one that is
"chemically and mechanically
nonirritating." When given in small, frequent
feedings, it may reduce symptoms caused by
narrowing or active inflammation in the
bowel. It is often unclear, however, which
foods should be included or excluded
because people differ in their food
tolerances. As a result, the bland diet should

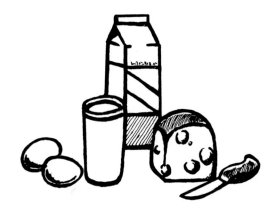

be individualized. Be guided by the food list
given by your physician or dietician.

The bland diet generally *excludes:*

- Spices and highly seasoned foods:
  Black and red pepper, chili powder,
  mustard, nutmeg. (Cinnamon, allspice,
  cloves, paprika and herbs usually do
  not produce symptoms.)
- Caffeine in coffee, tea, colas and the
  theobromine in chocolate.
- Alcohol
- Roughage: Especially raw fruits and
  vegetables with skins and small seeds,
  cereals and baked products made with
  unrefined flour, nuts, seeds, popcorn.

The Low-Residue/ Low-Fiber Diet

People with disease located in the terminal
ileum and/or colon may require what is
called a low-residue diet. A better name
might be a "low-roughage" diet, for the
dietary goal is to provide a minimum of
undigestable fiber that can block narrowed
intestinal areas or irritate an inflamed colon.
The problem is that the words *residue* and
fiber are used interchangeably, yet are not
really the same. Residue includes the total
feces made up of undigested and
unabsorbed food plus metabolic and
bacterial products. For example, milk and
prune juice contribute to fecal residue, yet

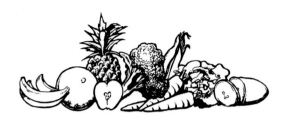

contain no fiber. Fiber is that portion of plants that is not digested by the human intestinal tract. There are several kinds of fiber: cellulose, hemicellulose, lignin, pectins and algal polysaccharides, each with different properties. Foods that are high in cellulose, hemicellulose, and lignin may have difficulty passing through narrowed areas or may cause irritation. This kind of fiber is often called ''roughage,'' hence the name ''low-roughage'' diet. Remember, the foods which come from animals do not contain fiber (roughage).

Foods Allowed:

Strict Low-Roughage Diet

Milk: Yogurt, cream

Cheese: Cottage, cream

Fats: Butter, margarine, vegetable oil, mayonnaise salad dressing.

Meat, poultry, fish: lean, tender beef, veal and lamb, chicken, turkey, fish (baked, boiled, broiled)

Soups: Broths, noodle and rice soups, creamed soups

Vegetables: Potatoes (boiled, mashed, baked, unseasoned vegetable juices in limited amounts)

Fruits: Clear fruit juices in limited amounts (grape, cranberry, apple, orange,* lemonade*)

Starches: Refined, enriched breads and cereals, macaroni, rice, noodles, spaghetti, crackers

(*if tolerated)

Desserts: Ices, ice cream*, pudding, custard,* gelatin, plain cake, candy and cookies without fruit or nuts

Beverages: Tea, coffee,* carbonated beverages

Condiments*: Salt and sugar, mild spices

Minimal-Roughage Diet

Milk: Yogurt, cream

Mild cheeses (e.g. cheddar, Swiss)

Fats: Butter, margarine, vegetable oil, mayonnaise salad dressing.

Meat, poultry, fish: lean, tender beef, veal and lamb, chicken, turkey, fish (baked, boiled, broiled)

Soups: Broths, noodle and rice soups, creamed soups, vegetable soups from those allowed

Potatoes plus cooked asparagus tips, green beans, spinach, squash, carrots, sweet potoatoes

Fruit juices, cooked or canned fruits without skins or seeds, ripe bananas

Starches: Refined, enriched breads and cereals, macaroni, rice, noodles, spaghetti, crackers

Desserts: Ices, ice cream,* pudding, custard,* gelatin, plain cake, candy and cookies without fruit or nuts

Beverages: Tea, coffee,* carbonated beverages

Condiments*: Salt and sugar, mild spices

The Low-Fat Diet

When Crohn's disease damages the ileum extensively, reabsorption of bile salts is greatly reduced. One important consequence of this is poor absorption of fats, fat soluble vitamins, calcium, and magnesium in the small intestine. A low-fat diet is often prescribed to help alleviate the symptoms caused by this situation.

Food Allowed:

Meats, Fish, Poultry
(baked, boiled, broiled)
Lean Beef
Lamb
Veal
Pork
Organ meats
Canadian bacon
Poultry—without skin
Low-fat fish and shellfish

Dairy:

Skim milk
Buttermilk
Low-fat and non-fat yogurt
Low-fat cheeses (Kraft® Naturals,
Churnley® brands)
Low-fat (1%) cottage cheese
Part-skim mozzarella
Special diet cheeses (Lite Line,®
Light & Lively®)

Soups:

Fat-free broth
Bouillon
Cream soups made with skim milk and
allowed meat and vegetables
Fat-free broths with meat, fish, poultry,
vegetables, rice, pasta added

Starches:

Breads, rolls
Pasta
Rice
Cereals of all kinds, except those with
oil and nuts (granolas)
Low fat pastries and cakes (many
brands now available)
Saltines, graham crackers
Vanilla wafers, ginger snaps, animal
crackers
(Avoid waffles, doughnuts, regular
pastries and coffee cakes)

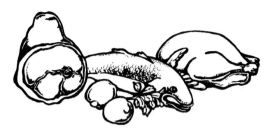

Fruits and Juices:

All kinds

Vegetables:

All except avocados

Desserts:

Sherbet
Fruit ice
Frozen low fat yogurt
Gelatin
Pudding made with skim milk
Angel food cake
Meringues
Clear soft and hard candies
Jelly
Jam
Syrup
Marshmallows
Not allowed:
Chocolate
Nuts
Ice Cream
Cake
Pie
Most cookies

Fats:

1–2 servings each meal
Example of 1 serving:
1 tsp. margarine, butter,
oil, mayonnaise
2 tbsp. half and half
2 tsp. peanut butter
1 strip crisp bacon
2 tsp. reduced fat,
margarine or salad dressing

Beverages:

  Coffee
  Tea
  Herb teas
  Carbonated beverages
  Cocoa made with skim milk
  Caffeine-free beverages
  Fruit juices
  Water

High-Protein/
High-Calorie Diet

A high-protein, high-calorie diet is frequently recommended to correct weight loss, to stimulate growth in growth-impaired children and adolescents, to replenish protein stores caused by intestinal loss, and to prevent deficiencies during treatment. Although an ideal goal, this diet is sometimes difficult to follow because of other dietary restrictions, such as fat or roughage. Choosing "nutrient-dense" foods—ones with the greatest nutrient/calorie ratios—can help fulfill calorie and nutrient goals. Happily, most Americans eat a very high protein diet, but unless calorie levels are adequate, the protein is used for energy rather than for the building of body tissue.

Diet Outline:

The daily diet plan should include the following foods or their nutritive equivalents in age-appropriate amounts:

  Milk: (whole) 4 servings (1 serving = 1 cup)
  Meat: (or meat substitutes) 2 large
    servings (1 serving = 3–4 ounces)
  Vegetables: (4 servings—including one
    green or yellow, one potato or
    substitute, and two others (1 serving =
    1/2 cup)
  Fruits: 3 servings—including one citrus
    (1 serving = 1/2 cup)

Enriched grains: 6 servings—including
    cereal, breads, pasta (1 serving = 1/2
    cup of pasta or 1 slice bread)
Fortified margarine or butter: 5 servings
Desserts and sweets: as desired

Supplemental formulas (listed in full-liquid diet) can be used with meals and snacks or in preparing soups, casseroles, desserts, milkshakes. Extra powdered milk can be added to creamed dishes, gravies, milk, cottage cheese, dips, peanut butter. Many extra calories can be provided by adding liberal amounts of butter, margarine or vegetable oil to appropriate foods. There are protein supplements with little lactose content that can be used similarly (Casec,® Propac,® Pro-mix®). Glucose and glucose polymers (e.g. Polycose,® Controlyte®) are less sweet than table sugar (sucrose) and can be used in larger amounts without making foods too sweet.

MCT oil contains almost 8 calories per cc.,(1 tsp = 5cc; 1 tbsp = 15 cc) and can be added in tiny amounts to many foods (soups, casseroles, sauces, desserts, milkshakes, juice), significantly increasing their caloric content. This oil is almost tasteless and less "oily" than other fats, but it does have two drawbacks. It can produce diarrhea when used in large amounts, and it is more expensive.

The high protein/high calorie diet is best implemented using small, frequent meals rather than large ones. Snacks become "meals" in their importance.

Protein Food Equivalents:

Each serving provides approximately 7 grams of protein. Fat and calorie values will vary.

Meats, poultry, fish (1 ounce portion):
  Eggs—1
  Canned fish—1/4 cup
  Sardines—3

Clams, oysters, shrimp, scallops—5
Cold cuts—1 slice (1/8 inch thick)
Hot dog—1

Nuts and Seeds:
(high-fiber, use with caution)
Almonds—25
Brazil nuts—10
Cashews—12–16
Peanuts or peanut butter—2 tbsp
Seeds—3 tbsp.

Dairy products:
Milk—1 cup
Yogurt—1 cup
Cheese—1 ounce (slice of most cheeses)
Grated parmesan—3 tbsp.
Cottage cheese—1/4 cup
Pudding, ice cream or sherbet, frozen
yogurt —1 (generous) cup
Legumes and lentils—
1/2 cup cooked
Tofu—1/3 cup
Grains
Bread—4 slices
Cereal—1 1/2 cups
Rice, potatoes, pasta—1 1/2 cups
cooked

Miscellaneous:
Pizza—1/8—10 inch pizza
Tacos—1/2
Macaroni and cheese 1/2–1 cup
Pot pie—1/2

*Vegetarians should check with their
physician and/or nutritionist to assure the
adequacy of their diets and correct
complimentary proteins.

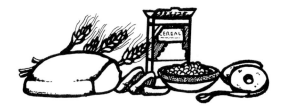

II. Rich Food Sources of Important Vitamins

Vitamin A:

Animal sources contain pre-formed
vitamin A:

Liver	Cheese
Eggs	Butter and Cream
Milk	Fish liver oils

Plant sources contain carotenes which
are converted to vitamin A in the body:

Dark green leafy vegetables:

Broccoli	Asparagus	Parsley
Spinach	Green peas	

Yellow vegetables and fruits:

Carrots	Sweet potatoes	
Peaches	Winter squash	Tomatoes
Oranges	Melons	

Vitamin D:

SUNLIGHT!
Liver
Fish liver oils
Fortified milk and milk powder
Butter and fortified margarines
Eggs
Fortified cereals (check labels)

Vitamin C (Ascorbic Acid):

Fruits	*Vegetables*
Citrus fruits	Broccoli
Strawberries	Tomatoes (raw),
Melons	tomato juice
Bananas	Dark green leafy
Apples	vegetables
	Cabbage
	Potatoes
	Green peppers
	Asparagus

Folic Acid (Folacin):

A special kind of anemia results from a deficiency of folic acid. This can occur when sulfasalazine interferes with its absorption. Supplemental folic acid is frequently given along with this medication. There are excellent food sources as well, but care must be taken in cooking and storage, for folic acid is easily destroyed by heat, light and air. The name folic acid or folacin is derived from the word "foliage," since green leafy vegetables are among its most important sources. Those on a restricted roughage diet can eat little "foliage," and will often be told to take a supplement, either as folic acid alone or else as part of a regular multivitamin, most of which contain at least 400 micrograms folic acid.

Foods Rich in Folic Acid (Folacin):

Liver	Green leafy vegetables:
Beets	Broccoli
Corn	Brussel sprouts
Frozen peas	Endive
Legumes and Lentils	Spinach
Parsnips	Romaine

Vitamin B-12:

Vitamin B-12 deficiency in IBD is commonly caused by ileal disease or resection of the ileum, the site of absorption of this vitamin It can also be the result of a vegetarian diet, since meat, fish and poultry are the principal dietary sources of this vitamin. Your physician will obtain serum levels periodically if you are in danger of becoming deficient and/or perform a Schilling Test to assess your ability to absorb vitamin B-12. True deficiency of this vitamin is usually treated by monthly levels in some individuals. Follow your physician's recommendations regarding which source is best for you.

III. Food Sources of Important Minerals

Calcium:

An adequate intake of calcium is important for everyone for strong bones and teeth. For the person with IBD, it is even more essential, because dietary restrictions may decrease the availability of this nutrient. Without milk in some form, it is difficult to get enough calcium, and supplements may be necessary. Check with your physician or nutritionist to find your requirement for calcium. Use the following table to combine foods that will provide that amount or ask to have a suitable supplement prescribed that will allow you to meet your need for calcium.

Foods Rich in Calcium:

The following foods contain 300 milligrams of calcium:

Milk: All kinds (skim, whole, buttermilk)—1 cup
Dry Skim Milk Powder—1/3 cup
Yogurt: 1 cup
Sardines: 3 ounces

The following foods contain 200 milligrams of calcium:

Cheese: American, cheddar, brick, processed cheese food—1 ounce
Ice cream or ice milk: (Regular kinds)—1 cup
(Richer ice creams—e.g. Baskin Robbins® contain only 100 mg per cup.)
Cheese souffle: 1 serving ($3\frac{1}{4}$" × $3\frac{1}{4}$" × 2")
Cooked greens: 1 cup

The following foods contain 150 milligrams of calcium:

Pudding: All kinds (made from mixes, rice, bread)—1/2 cup
Baked custard: 1/2 cup
Pizza: 1 serving (¼ of 10" diameter cheese pizza, ¼" thick)
Cream soup made with milk: Tomato, chicken, asparagus, etc.—1 cup

The following foods contain 100 milligrams of calcium:

Cheese: all kinds—1 cubic inch
Cottage cheese: 1/2 cup
Creamed Chicken: 1 cup
Rich ice cream: (Baskin-Robbins® type) 1 cup
Custard pie: (1/6 pie) 1 serving
Dried beans: (cooked) 1 cup
Peanuts: 1 cup
Frozen yogurt

Miscellaneous Foods:
Eggs: 1 large—30 mg
Bread: 1 slice—20 mg
Nuts, dried beans and vegetable greens contain large amounts of calcium, but it is in a form which is not readily used by the body.

Iron:

Many people with IBD are frequently anemic. There are a number of possible causes for this, and anemia cannot usually be treated with diet alone. Iron supplements are necessary, but can cause bowel irritation and cramping. It is therefore helpful to have some information about ways to increase the amount of iron in the food we eat. There are two kinds of iron in food—heme and non-heme iron. Heme iron is found in red meat. Non-heme iron is found mostly in plant foods and is less available to the body. Eating non-heme iron foods with meat, fish or poultry will increase its absorption.

Eating a food rich in vitamin C will also increase the absorption of both heme and non-heme iron. This information will allow you to plan meals that will enhance the absorption and availability of the iron in all your foods.

Iron Equivalents:
Each serving of the foods listed below yields approximately 1 milligram of iron.
Liver: 1/2 ounce
Beef: 1 ounce
Egg: 1
Chicken: 3 ounces
Legumes and lentils: 1/3 cup cooked
Greens: 1/3 cup (including spinach)
Potatoes: 1 medium
Rice, spaghetti, noodles:
Prunes: 4
Raisins: 1/6 cup
Pork, lamb: 1 ounce
Hot dogs: 1 (8 per pound)
Oysters: 1 medium
Fish: (Fresh, canned tuna, sardines, salmon)—3 oz.
Fishsticks: 10
Most fruits: 1 cup
Most breads: 2 slices
Many prepared cereals: 1 oz. (Check labels)
Milk: 10 cups

Zinc:

It has been suggested that zinc deficiency may have a role in IBD, and that zinc supplementation might be considered in its treatment, especially in children with growth impairment. While the role of zinc in IBD is still unclear, it is important as a component of many enzymes in the body and it plays an essential role in DNA and RNA synthesis.

Zinc deficiency can be produced by malabsorption and increased intestinal losses. Foods high in fiber can also interfere with its absorption. In addition, zinc, iron and copper can compete with each other for incorporation into compounds in the body. For this reason the *ratio* of these metals to each other is very sensitive, and supplementation should be undertaken *only* with the advice of your physician and/or nutritionist.

Food Rich in Zinc:

Animal Foods
  Beef, lamb, pork veal
  Chicken, turkey (dark meat)
  Liver, heart
  Crab, lobster, oysters, shrimp
  Cheese (cheddar, American, gouda,
    mozzarella, muenster, Swiss)

Plant Foods
  Legumes and lentils
  Bran
  Nuts
  Green peas
  Grains (wheat, rice, wheat germ and
    products made from these)

Summary

Deficiencies of essential nutrients may occur in IBD depending on the location and extent of disease. The primary nutrients are: protein, calories, vitamins A, D, C, B-12 and folic acid; calcium, iron, and zinc. No doubt, other deficiencies occur. The best protection is to eat a variety of foods from the basic four food groups, choosing sources that are rich in the nutrients you need and that conform to the dietary modifications you require.

Sometimes vitamin and/or mineral supplements are needed for optimal health. Be guided by the advice of your physician or nutritionist in your choice of supplements.

IBD and Your Self-Image

17

Having a chronic illness affects *every* aspect of a person's life—from attending school and holding a job to relating to family and friends and establishing intimate relationships. How we manage to cope in each of these areas depends very much on how we look at ourselves, in other words, on our self-image. Do we view the additional burden imposed by IBD as proof that we will fail at these important life tasks? Or is IBD only a "footnote" to a life filled with the rewards of friendship, love, and meaningful activity?

Symptoms like pain, diarrhea, fever and weakness invariably assault our self-confidence and prevent us from recognizing our strengths.

Of course, how we feel about ourselves depends on how physically sick we are and whether we are able to engage in our usual activities. Symptoms like pain, diarrhea, fever and weakness, in addition to the effects of medications like corticosteroids, invariably assault our self-confidence and prevent us from recognizing our strengths, attractiveness, and endearing qualities.

To help IBD sufferers in dealing with these critical issues, we asked psychotherapist **Audrey Kron** to answer some of the questions people ask most about IBD and self-image. Kron has experienced Crohn's disease for more than 30 years (See story in Chapter 15). She is the Director of the Center for Coping with Chronic Illness and on the staff at Hutzel Hospital in Detroit. As psychological liaison for the Michigan Chapter of CCFA, she originated their Coping Conference and writes the "Ask Audrey" column for their newsletter.

Question: Since I have had Crohn's disease, I have experienced so many different feelings that I'm beginning to wonder if I'm abnormal. Please let me know if others also experience mood swings.

Answer: With the onset of an illness such as inflammatory bowel disease, there are many different emotional states that are quite common and predictable. Each individual is different, but there are some difficult feelings we all share:

- *Fear.* There may be fears about how the illness will affect work, school, or the future in general. Some of us worry that we will lose the love of our family and friends. Others are afraid of possible pain, side effects from medications, hospitalization, and testing procedures.
- *Anger.* "Why Me?" is a common question. Sometimes the anger is directed against fate, but often it gets displaced onto the people closest to us: family and friends.
- *Guilt.* Even though we do not know the cause of these diseases, we may feel that we have done something to contribute to the onset of the illness. Even if that's not a concern, there may be guilty feelings for the extra burden that illness imposes on the family.
- *Shame.* In our society, we hide anything that has to with the bathroom, so people with IBD often feel shame because they have a disease that has to do with the bowels.
- *Depression.* At times it seems like everything is going wrong. Life seems overwhelming and it seems hard to realize that things *will* get better.

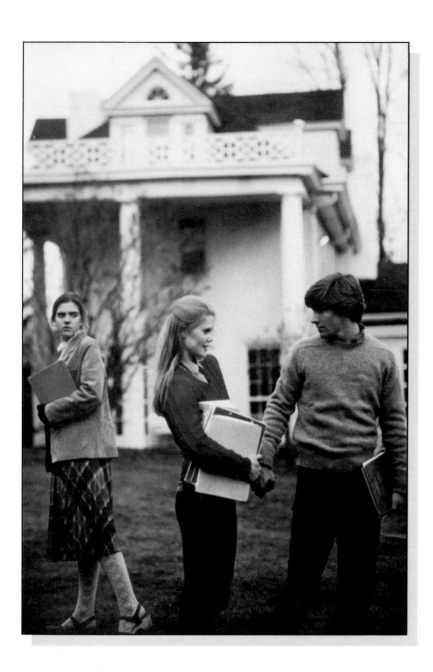

- *Frustration.* Sometimes our bodies do not react in the way that we would like. We find we can't do all the things we'd prefer. It's easy to become frustrated.
- *Alienation.* There are times when we feel very alone. It seems like no one can understand what we are feeling.

None of these feelings are abnormal. The important thing is to recognize that there are many uncomfortable feelings that we will experience. If we can recognize these feelings, we will be able to talk to others about them. This is an important part of the process of learning to accept them.

Question: How do you make and keep friends with an illness like IBD? Sometimes I find it easier to just not see people.

Answer: Friends are very important, especially so if you have a chronic illness. There are many ways to make and maintain friendships despite the limitations of IBD. Let's look at some of them:

Friends want to help you but not knowing how, they may say nothing and just not call or come around. Your communication skills will have to be better. Learning how to share feelings often opens the way for further communication. Asking friends to do a small task can relieve their sense of helplessness. You may need a ride to the doctor, a dinner brought in, or just a phone call or visit. It makes them feel better to do something specific and concrete for you.

It's tempting when something is hurting you to tell everybody all the details. Others may be interested for a while, but they become uncomfortable when you elaborate too often. If every time they ask you "How do you feel?," you say, "My stomach hurts," etc., eventually they'll stop asking. It is important to be able to share these feelings with some people, but be selective. Make sure they really want to hear. You cannot blame people for not wanting to be around if your digestive system is the only topic of conversation.

When you are invited somewhere, instead of saying "I can't go," make the situation one you can handle. Sometimes things like checking out the bathroom, making special arrangements for food, being dropped off at the door, etc. can be just what is needed to make you comfortable. Learn to accept the limitations of your friends. Nobody's perfect! If we are looking for acceptance from friends, we have to be able to offer it as well.

Question: I'm having a difficult time finding dates, let alone a marriage partner. Do people with IBD date, get married and have normal family lives?

Answer: Of course, people with IBD can have normal family lives. However, it is common to hear of single people with IBD, young and old alike, who feel that nobody would want them.

The first thing to do is to ask yourself: "Would I be a desirable mate *without* my IBD?" If I don't like myself, nobody else will. What are my strong points? Do I have a good sense of humor? Am I a caring person? Do I listen and speak well? Am I intelligent? Do I have good common sense?

The list is endless, and if we really think about it, each of us has many strong points that can be enhanced. It's important to do the best with what we have, and it's always amazing to learn what others find attractive. Sometimes physical features that we consider a liability can actually be an asset. Even the illness can affect others in diverse ways. One person may find it overwhelming, another, a challenge. What is of prime importance is how we feel about ourselves.

The partner who accepts you with the illness is someone who loves you in spite of it.

Quality of Life in IBD: What Does the Research Say?

René Dubois once described quality of life as deriving "profound satisfaction from the activities of daily life." For the person with IBD, difficulties in coping with unpredictable and painful symptoms, nutritional depletion, frequent hospitalization and surgery can severely compromise the carrying out of daily activities. Interestingly, although there is no evidence of a causal relationship between psychological factors and either disease, a recent study found that half of Crohn's disease patients and one quarter of ulcerative colitis patients studied suffered from some form of emotional problem, usually depression. This is not surprising, given the debilitating nature of the diseases. What is more surprising is that most quality of life studies have found that people with IBD are functioning well despite their compromised health status.

A 1985 study of 85 British outpatients with Crohn's disease found that most were able to work and enjoyed supportive personal relationships, despite a somewhat diminished interest in sexual activity. However, another British study in the same year found that of 84 people with ulcerative colitis, one fifth had a reduced earning capacity and had problems dealing with bowel symptoms before or during working hours. A fear of incontinence caused many to limit or curtail social activities. Similarly, a Danish population-based study found that while people with Crohn's disease did not differ markedly from other people in their social and working patterns, 54 percent of them felt that their illness placed a strain on their personal and working lives.

(Continued on next page.)

(Continued from previous page)

Although surgery cures ulcerative colitis, patients with Crohn's disease must undergo operation *without* the reassurance that the disease will not recur. Nevertheless, a 1980 study of 51 patients after their first operation for Crohn's disease found that despite disease recurrence or creation of an ileostomy, 92 percent felt that surgery had improved the quality of their lives. In a recent national survey of the CCFA membership, **Dr. Douglas A. Drossman** and his co-workers at the University of North Carolina found that ostomates with ulcerative colitis and even those with Crohn's disease have as good as or better quality of life than patients who have not had this operation.

The picture that emerges from these studies is that people with IBD generally go on with life's activities despite frequent interruptions by disease and its treatments. This is particularly true of the recent CCFA study. Dr. Drossman, the study's principal author, cautions that because Foundation members benefit from education and psychological support, they may not be typical of most people with IBD. However, several studies including the CCFA study, point out that the long-term outlook is considerably bleaker for those with onset of IBD in childhood or adolescence. These young patients, particularly those with Crohn's disease, have more hospitalizations, more surgery, longer exposure to toxic medications, more complications, and more overall dysfunction than older patients.

Now suppose you are doing everything you can to make yourself a desirable partner and taking part in activities to meet people, but you still run into disappointment. Perhaps you've found someone who won't accept your illness. Unfortunately, there are some people who want perfection in their partners. You should feel lucky to find this out ahead of time. These are the people who wouldn't be able to deal with any of the normal kinds of problems that come up during a marriage, including illness. They probably would have a hard time dealing with a mate who became less attractive, or coping with the inevitable aging process.

On the other hand, the partner who accepts you *with* the illness is someone who loves you in spite of it. With such a person, you have a much better chance of making the marriage work. So instead of worrying about finding someone, find yourself, make yourself strong, and someone who can fully appreciate your strengths will find you.

Question: What kinds of sexual problems do people with IBD experience?

Answer: The simple answer to your question is that IBD does *not* stand in the way of a very satisfactory sex life. However, there are areas that could cause problems:

- *General symptoms of the illness.* This is the most common culprit with IBD patients. Pain, fatigue, nausea, or diarrhea all can impede your sex life when you are experiencing these symptoms. However, with good communication and some planning, these problems *can* be overcome. Fatigue can certainly put a damper on sexual activity. But, with a little planning, it's possible to find the times when you feel the strongest. It's hard to think about sex when you are in pain (although you may find that sex can divert attention away from the pain), but the way you handle it is very important. Here's where communication plays an important role. Love, caring and sexuality can be expressed in many ways besides intercourse. You know how. Sometimes, it's easy to forget.

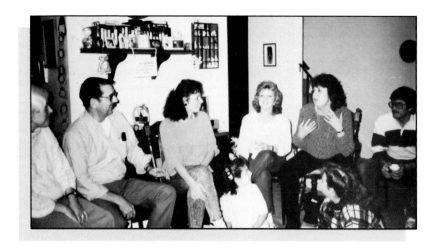

A CCFA support group in action.

- *The psychological impact of the illness.* Sexual relations are strained when we feel depressed or concerned about our body image, or our role in the family or at work. Any progress or difficulty in these areas will usually show up in the bedroom. Communication, again, is the key word. How we look, how we speak, how we act and most of all, how we feel can all contribute to our sexual attractiveness.

Some of us fear that we will be unattractive if we have to have an ostomy. This can stimulate fears of abandonment. Ostomy surgery need not interfere with sexual activity (See Chapter 6). Again, a person who loves you won't be bothered, and why would you bother with a person who didn't love you?

- *Specific fears about sex and IBD.* People with IBD may fear that sexual activity will provoke symptoms, or that sex life cannot be resumed after surgery. Some fear that sex will make the illness worse. Some fear pregnancy.

Another less serious but more embarrassing problem is the possibility of having an accident during intercourse. True, it can be embarrassing, but remember that your partner loves you and is more concerned about *your* reaction. How you handle the situation makes a great deal of difference.

In all situations, it's important to focus on your potential, and not on your limitations. Realize that sexual feelings are expressed in many ways.

How Can a Support Group Help You to Cope?

If you have never joined a support group (or self-help group) for people with IBD, you may be wondering how such a group can help you. What do people talk about in a support group? How do people find enough to say to others they may never have met before?

Most CCFA chapters around the country sponsor self-help groups. Here is a sampling of topics used by groups in some CCFA chapters:

1. **Reaction to Having a Chronic Illness:** What does it feel like to find out, perhaps half-way through life, that you have a chronic illness? How did you find out, what were your early symptoms? Was there a long delay in your diagnosis?

2. **Reaction of Friends and Family:** Who is your support system? Is it a parent, spouse, sibling, friend? How did these people react when you were first diagnosed? Were you given erroneous advice from friends and well-wishers about the nature of your illness? (Many group members may have been told their disease was due to stress or poor eating habits, etc.) Is it easy to ask for help when you need it? How do family and friends react to long bouts or flare-ups?

3. **Impact of IBD on Lifestyle:** Can you work, go to school, take a vacation, go out with friends? Have you missed work days or classes? If you are single, can you have a social life that is normal? Are there certain precautions you take if you know you will be taking a long car ride not knowing where the next bathroom may be? Does your life depend on where the bathroom is? Can you be open about that need or must it be a secret?

(Continued on next page)

Flexibility, communication, understanding, and humor are all important tools in finding sexual fulfillment.

Question: What do I do about friends and family members who leave me out of social activities and responsibilities because of my IBD? I don't want any special treatment and I certainly don't want to be left out.

Answer: Often family and friends feel that they are being helpful by protecting us. What they don't realize is that they are diminishing us as individuals by not letting us make decisions for ourselves. Sometimes others feel that because we are having troubles with our body that we are also intellectually compromised as well. It's important to explain to family and friends what it is that we feel. We have to tell them that it's important for us to retain our sense of autonomy. Regardless of whether we can or cannot do something, it is important to us to be consulted on matters affecting our lives.

We too, have to take some responsibility. We have to let others know what we can do and how we plan on doing it. We have to learn to say no to things that we feel we cannot handle, and find creative ways to deal with the obligations that we do take on. Talk with the significant people in your life and let them know that you want the option of deciding for yourself what you can and cannot do.

Question: Sometimes things get to be too much to handle on my own. How do I know when it's time to get professional help?

Answer: Many people handle the challenges that come with IBD on their own. Others benefit from the encouragement and camaraderie of a support group. When should you seek individual counseling? Feelings of anger, guilt, resentment, depression or lack of self-esteem can all be indications that therapy could be helpful. Here is a simple rule to follow: If you are unhappy with the way things are and you feel that you can't do anything about it, it may be time to see a professional. The main purpose of therapy is to help you understand what's keeping you from accomplishing what you desire.

Chronic illness can create problems in a relationship or intensify problems that existed before the onset of the illness. You may need short-term therapy to help you to get through a difficult period or intensive therapy to solve a persistent problem. The therapist should understand the nature of IBD and the drugs used to treat it. He/she should maintain a close working relationship with your physician. In fact, your gastroenterologist may be able to recommend a suitable psychotherapist who is knowledgeable about IBD and about what you are going through.

Chronic illness can create many problems, but it also creates effective problem-solvers: people who are accustomed to overcoming obstacles every day of their lives. Knowing when to ask for help is not a sign of weakness but a sign of strength. It means that you are unwilling to let your illness keep you from enjoying all the richness that life has to offer.

(Continued from previous page)

4. **Dealing with Your Physician:** Is your doctor available to you? Does he/she answer all your questions or do you feel he/she may be holding information back? Does your doctor tell you about the possible side-effects of your medication or spend time with you on the phone?

5. **Feelings about Medical Treatment:** How do you feel about surgery, tests, having to take medications such as prednisone? What are the effects of prednisone on your mood, your appearance, the way you feel about yourself? How do you feel about trying new medications?

6. **Feelings about Sex:** Do you have fears about something happening during sexual intercourse (particularly with single people), fears of being unattractive, fears about having children? How open can you be with a prospective mate without scaring him/her off? How do you explain the side-effects of medication to a friend or mate?

7. **Using the Illness:** Is it possible to use your illness to get attention or pity? Is it a way to cop out when necessary? Do sick youngsters get more attention from their parents? How does that create problems in the family? When is psychotherapy a good idea?

8. **Sharing Coping Strategies:** Is it a good idea to carry an extra change of underwear at all times, or a portable toilet in the car, or to check ahead to find where the bathrooms are located? Should you talk to teachers on behalf of a child to make sure of immediate access to toilet facilities, etc.?

Physical Activity and IBD

18

P hysical exercise and participation in sports are just as important for people with inflammatory bowel disease as they are for everyone. There is usually some physical activity that a person with IBD can master and enjoy despite the limitations of illness. The choice of which physical activity/sport to participate in is highly personal, of course. Even the less active sports, such as golf and bowling, can provide a sense of achievement as well as the benefits of social interaction.

The Benefits of Aerobic Activity

The past few decades have seen an explosion in the participation of people all over the world in physical activity. The popularization of aerobics has given a strong impetus to that development. **Aerobics** is defined as activity that increases the work of the heart to a submaximal level while the body's oxygen demands are supplied by a greater intake of air from the lungs. One should be able to continue to talk while engaging in aerobic activity.

Aerobic physical activity, such as fast walking, jogging, swimming, cycling, and rowing, tends to reverse muscle weakness and wasting, and prevent calcium and protein loss from bone; some or all of these problems may occur in IBD. Numerous studies have shown that people who take the time to engage in aerobic exercise feel a sense of well-being and accomplishment. There is a psychological ''high'' achieved during prolonged aerobics, possibly because of the release of special hormones in the brain called **endorphins.** The endorphins appear to lift the spirits, especially during periods of depression, help to erase negative feelings about the body, and even relieve pain.

All studies report an increased sense of well-being among those who do exercise.

The failure to exercise may have negative effects on the body's resistance to disease. A recent study has shown that college athletes who did not maintain their physical fitness were at higher risk from coronary artery disease than were college nonathletes who later entered an aerobic program and became fit. Other studies have demonstrated that sedentary people have a higher mortality rate from coronary artery disease than active people, even those who only engage in mild activity, such as walking. Although no research has shown that people who exercise *actually live longer,* all studies report an increased sense of well-being among those who do exercise.

The lesson here is that all people, even those with a chronic disease like IBD, can always find *some* physical activity to enjoy despite certain restrictions and precautions they might have to take. This activity is likely to improve general health (especially the activity of the heart and lungs) and psychological health as well.

Exercise and the Gastrointestinal Tract

Although there is still very little information about the effects of exercise on gastrointestinal function, we have learned a few important facts during the past decade. During exercise, secretion of stomach acid is decreased and blood flow to the intestinal tract is also decreased, sometimes by as

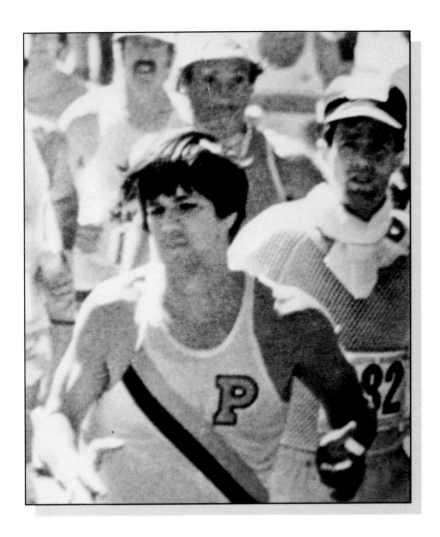

much as 80 percent. These changes do not appear to affect the absorption of food. There is still debate about whether the stomach empties at a faster or slower rate with exercise. Stomach emptying appears to be more rapid at low levels and much slower at intense levels of physical activity. Heartburn caused by acid backing up into the esophagus is a problem for long-distance runners. It is also likely that food moves more slowly through the small intestine during physical exercise.

The most common gastrointestinal complaints noted during prolonged aerobic exercise, particularly running or other "bouncy" sports, are an increased urge to move the bowels, cramps, diarrhea, nausea and vomiting. These problems occur much less often in sports where the body is relatively stable, such as cycling, swimming, skating or cross country skiing. Not everyone who excercises will experience these problems; they may even decrease the more the body gets used to aerobic activity.

Nutrition, Fluids and Exercise

Everyone needs an adequate supply of calories as well as appropriate amounts of carbohydrates (sugars), fats, proteins, fluids, vitamins, calcium, potassium and trace elememts to maintain life and health. During prolonged physical activity, energy is derived first from glycogen (carbohydrates that are stored in muscle). Later, energy is released from the breakdown of fats; if fats are unavailable, the body then breaks down protein to supply its energy needs. For this reason, carbohydrates, especially complex carbohydrates, should be the main component of the diet, since they take longer to break down compared to simple carbohydrates.

Fats are an essential part of the diet and should be of the poly-unsaturated or mono-unsaturated variety. Proteins are needed for growth and maintenance of body tissues. The body's need for protein rises with increased physical activity, with fever and infection, and with increased protein losses from severe diarrhea.

During exercise, the person with IBD may be more susceptible to problems involving fluid loss than at other times. The following general suggestions are important to follow:

1. Avoid eating solid foods for three hours before any aerobic exercise.
2. Take liquid foods as pre-exercise meals and during exercise; these liquids should not include fats and proteins.
3. Whenever fluid intake is a first priority, the drink should be low in carbohydrates.
4. Large amounts of body fluids are lost during exercise, especially if the person exercising has diarrhea or an ileostomy. Drink copious amounts of fluids both *before* and *after* aerobic exercise and realize that it may not be enough to rely on thirst alone when deciding to replace lost fluids. *Drinking during exercise should be part of any training program.*
5. Fluids can be simply water, commercial preparations such as Gatorade, or a combination of glucose with fructose (fruit sugar).
6. Vitamins are often lost by people with IBD, especially those taking steroids. Potassium supplements or foods high in potassium may need to be replaced if you experience frequent diarrhea while exercising.

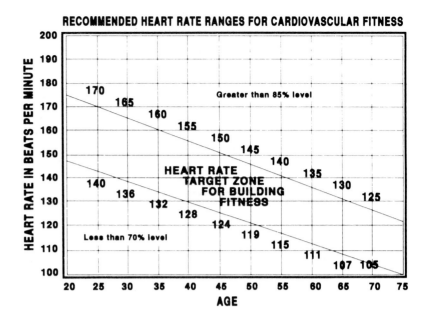

RECOMMENDED HEART RATE RANGES FOR CARDIOVASCULAR FITNESS

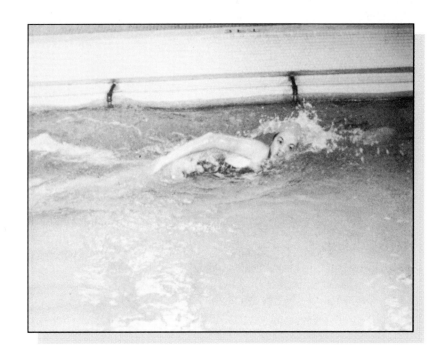

Which Sport is Best for Me?

While you may choose any sport you wish, some sports are less likely to stimulate gastrointestinal problems than others, and some may pose fewer risks to you as a person with IBD. You will remember that "gliding" aerobic sports such as cycling seem to produce fewer gastrointestinal symptoms than "bouncy" sports, such as running. Active sports can be grouped into four categories: (1) nonaerobic sports (golf, tennis, bowling); (2) weight training; (3) contact sports; (4) endurance (aerobic) sports. We have already noted the benefits of nonaerobic sports for the person with IBD. Weight training, using free weights or machines such as the Nautilus or Universal, can be helpful in rebuilding certain muscle groups that have become weakened by disease or by the use of corticosteroids. Patients with Crohn's disease have demonstrated how weight training can overcome the weakness caused by their illness. We suggest that you contact your gastroenterologist or a physical therapist before starting weight training, since this type of activity has been known occasionally to increase bowel symptoms. If you notice any increase in your symptoms, you should discontinue this type of activity.

Contact sports such as football may expose the person with IBD to a greater risk for injury than others, especially if bones have been weakened by prolonged bedrest, calcium depletion or steroids, or if there has been ostomy surgery. But there are many exceptions and Rolf Benirschke and Uwe von Schamann, both ulcerative colitis sufferers, continued to play professional football using proper precautions. Most recently, Kevin Dineen has demonstrated his outstanding ability as a hockey player while still suffering from Crohn's disease (See story).

Endurance or aerobic sports, such as jogging, cycling, swimming, or rowing, cause no physical contact, and therefore pose less chance of injury. As noted, in addition to improving cardiovascular performance they will help you to achieve a sense of well-being because of their ability to stimulate the release of endorphins in the brain. Together with your physician, you should select the sports and activities that will be most helpful physically and psychologically in maintaining your health.

Maintaining body fluids is more difficult for people with IBD since they normally lose fluids faster because of frequent loose stools or ostomy discharge.

The Person with IBD

Certain conditions characteristic of IBD may have a bearing on which type of activities you should avoid, or what special precautions you must take to allow for safer participation in sports. Perianal disease such as fissures, fistulas, and abscesses might obviously be aggravated during activities such as horseback riding, biking and perhaps even running. It would be wise to avoid such activities when these complications are active.

Maintaining body fluids is more difficult for people with IBD since they normally lose fluids faster because of frequent loose stools or ostomy discharge. Since dehydration contributes to the increased incidence of renal stones, remember to drink lots of fluids before, during and after exercise. If you feel lightheaded and more tired than you should after exercise, or if you have muscle cramps or a marked decrease in the amount of urine you pass, you are probably not drinking enough fluids. Sometimes, taking an antidiarrheal medication like Imodium®

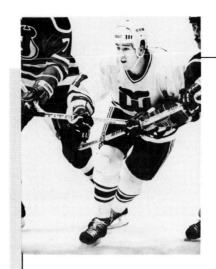

Kevin Dineen

"When I first found out that I had Crohn's disease, I kept it to myself," says Kevin Dineen, who plays for the Hartford Whalers hockey team. Diagnosed in 1987, Dineen at first ignored his illness. "I treated Crohn's like any other injury," he recalls. "I didn't want the disease to get in my way. Looking back now, that wasn't very smart."

After several flare-ups, Dineen learned to "respect" the disease: "I had to change my lifestyle. That meant eating the right foods and knowing when to relax and take it easy." Tough and aggressive on the ice despite Crohn's disease, Kevin Dineen has earned praise from teammates and is one of the best and most respected players in the National Hockey League.

or Lomotil® before exercise may help to prevent exercise-induced diarrhea.

Painful joints (knees, hips, ankles) may cause you to modify or stop physical activity. Treatment with nonsteroidal anti-inflammatory medications, such as Advil,® Motrin,® Naprosyn,® may be helpful, but there is evidence that these drugs and others like them can cause gastrointestinal bleeding and may aggravate the symptoms of IBD. The use of any anti-inflammatory medications should be discussed first with your gastroenterologist.

Anemia is common in many people with IBD. It may be caused by a folic acid deficiency, by inadequate amounts of iron in the diet, or by excessive loss of iron in the stool. Red blood cells are necessary to carry oxygen to tissue and this need obviously increases during exercise. Therefore, people with anemia need to raise their blood count to as near normal as possible, especially if strenuous exercise is planned. Check with your doctor about which supplements are best for you. Long distance running itself may induce a slight anemia because of the loss of small amounts of blood in the GI tract; periodic blood counts of runners with IBD is a good idea.

Steroids cause fluid retention, weak muscles, soft bones, and easily bruisable skin. Calcium and potassium are also lost when steroids are taken for long periods. If you are taking steroids and notice muscle cramps, spasms, skin bruising, bone or joint pain during physical activity, you should report this immediately to your physician. You may need both a change in your IBD treatment and a change in your exercise program. On the other hand, aerobic sports that exercise the long bones can actually *increase* the density of calcium in bones weakened by previous corticosteroid treatment.

Before beginning your exercise program, consult your physician. Your physician is responsible for coordinating a medical treatment program and will know why any exercise program should or should not be started. It is also a good idea to consult experts in exercise training or sports medicine or a physical therapist if there is any muscle, joint or bone injury. Many medical centers now have pain programs or ''beginning exercises'' for people with specific medical problems.

Traveling with IBD

19

All of us enjoy our freedom to travel within the United States and abroad, IBD sufferers no less than others. The IBD sufferer cannot leave illness at home along with the pets, so plans have to be made and answers prepared to the question "what if . . . ?"

Traveling within the United States

The United States, with its enormous geographical and climatic contrast, offers wonderful opportunities for travel and exploration which many of us tend to overlook. For travelers who have IBD, there is the comfortable knowledge that the drinking water throughout the country is pure and that the risks of traveler's diarrhea and food poisoning are remote. There should also be no problem with regard to health insurance coverage and there is a national standard of treatment for the complications of IBD if a flare-up of symptoms should occur.

Before traveling within the U.S., however, it is a good idea to discuss your plans with your physician to be sure that you are fit enough to make your planned trip. You should take with you enough current medication to last the length of the trip. Take along your physician's telephone number in your wallet so that you can contact his/her office in any sort of emergency. Also be sure to carry your insurance card, just in case. Let your doctor know where in particular you plan to visit, as he/she can often give you the name of a colleague in that part of the country. Doctors who treat IBD usually know good reliable physicians in every part of the country who would be able to handle any type of IBD emergency. If your case is particularly complex, it would be wise for your doctor to give you a typed summary describing your history, physical findings and current medications.

Doctors who treat IBD usually know good reliable physicians in every part of the country who would be able to handle any type of IBD emergency.

These comments also apply to travel to Canada, Bermuda, Puerto Rico and the U.S. Virgin Islands. However, if you plan to travel to Canada or Bermuda, check with your insurance carrier just to be sure that medical expenses are covered if the need were to arise.

Travel by car and camper is easy and generally poses few problems. Likewise, bus and train travel are relatively comfortable. Remember to find out in advance if the tour bus has a toilet. Long air trips, such as coast-to-coast or to Hawaii, can be tiring. It is always a good plan to try to get an aisle seat, so make arrangements ahead of time with the airline. Airlines are very helpful with special diets, but they need a few days prior notification of your needs.

If you plan any really vigorous or new exercise such as skiing or hiking in the National Parks, discuss this with your doctor and be sure that you know your own limits. Any back-packing trip where medical care is unavailable should be seriously discussed before you make final plans.

Overseas Travel and Travel to Latin America

Foreign travel demands fairly careful planning not only for your trip, but also for the possibility of trouble with your IBD.

Travel to Western Europe, Scandinavia, most of Eastern Europe, Australia, New Zealand and South Africa carries little risk of exposure to unpleasant illness. Travel to Latin America, the Caribbean and less developed countries does have its risks, especially if you leave the standard "tourist circuit." Cruises rarely expose you to any illness worse than sunburn and weight gain! However, it is wise to inquire in advance about the medical facilities available on board the ship.

Travel to the tropics often requires special immunizations, so again check with your doctor long before you leave on a trip. Find out about the risk of malaria, which is unfortunately making a major comeback in Africa and Asia. Hepatitis can be a risk in the developing countries as well as in the Mediterranean, so injections against hepatitis A and B may be recommended. Next, contact your medical insurance carrier and find out if there are forms to complete to keep up your coverage when you are out of the U.S.

After you have carried out these preliminary steps, you must get down to your basic medical needs for the trip. Make sure you have all your medications in their appropriate vials, properly labelled. Customs officers can be very suspicious when faced with pills not contained in vials with your name on them, so keep all medicines in separate individuals vials. Do not take samples and try not to use any type of pill box, except for use on the plane. Always carry your medications with you through customs. Do not check them in with your baggage! If you need narcotic medications, such as tincture of opium or codeine tablets,

Diarrhea afflicts one out of three U.S. travelers to less developed countries.

be doubly certain that the bottle or vial is labelled and that the label is secure. Let your pharmacist know that you will be taking your medicines out of the country.

How to Keep Healthy When Traveling

Diarrhea afflicts one out of three U.S. travelers to less developed countries. The odds are in your favor that you won't come down with "turista," "Delhi belly," or "Montezuma's revenge." However, there are guidelines which will cut down on the risk of contracting diarrhea, which is usually caused by an organism such as enterotoxigenic (entero = intestinal, toxi = toxin or poison, genic = producing) *Escherichia coli*. This organism is passed to travelers by fecal contamination of water or food. The guidelines are:

- Avoid tap water and all beverages containing water served in a pitcher. Water that has been boiled thoroughly (such as for tea) is acceptable, as are commercially bottled beverages. Be sure to open all bottles yourself or have them opened in your presence to be sure that tap water is not added.
- Avoid all ice and ice cream.
- Avoid all raw vegetables and salads.
- Avoid uncooked dairy products such as milk and cheese unless you are sure that they are pasteurized and prepared under sterile conditions.
- Never eat food from vendor's carts.
- Never eat prepared foods such as potato salad and cocktail canapes— even in elegant surroundings.
- Peel all fruits yourself.
- Peel egg shells yourself.

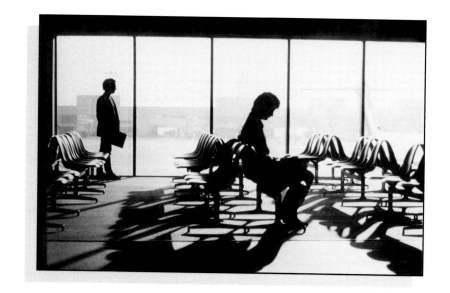

Most resort and business hotels in lesser developed countries have special water purification equipment, but always check with hotel staff to find out about their facilities. When in doubt, stick to bottled mineral water, even when you brush your teeth. Bath water may not be purified, so don't swallow water when showering. Be careful when swimming in fresh water, in dubious swimming pools, or where the ocean may be polluted.

There are two schools of thought about taking medicine to prevent traveler's diarrhea. A recent National Institutes of Health consensus development panel recommended that in healthy individuals the risk of using preventive medication outweighs the benefits, and that antimicrobial medicines are better used for *treatment* of traveler's diarrhea than for prevention. The other opinion would offer preventive medicines to those who would like to take them after careful consideration of possible side effects.

The IBD patient has to be given special consideration since a two to four-day bout with diarrhea may be very unpleasant and demoralizing. Small doses of the antibiotic doxycycline have been effective in preventing diarrhea in U.S. citizens traveling abroad and the cheaper antimicrobial trimethoprim, with or without sulfamethoxazole, is also effective. (Patients taking sulfasalazine would be wise to *avoid* taking the trimethoprim and sulfonamide combination.) These drugs are also effective in treating diarrhea, as is Pepto Bismol® in very large doses. Cipro® has recently become the drug of choice for many gastroenterologists, since it is effective against a broad spectrum of illnesses.

Gastroenterologists differ in their advice to IBD patients about taking any of the above medicines to protect against traveler's diarrhea, so each person with IBD should discuss this carefully with his/her doctor.

Danger Signals for the Traveler with IBD

- **High fever and shaking chills.** This could represent a systemic bacterial inflammation requiring intravenous antibiotic therapy.
- **Profuse bloody diarrhea.** This would suggest marked ulceration of the intestines either by a bacterium, parasite, or a major flare-up of colitis.
- **Severe abdominal pain and/or abdominal distension.** This could represent a complication of IBD, especially if associated with severe abdominal tenderness or nausea and vomiting.
- **Dizziness on standing up or an episode of fainting.** This could have several meanings. One is dehydration causing a lowering of blood pressure and requiring intravenous rehydration. Another is ''adrenal insufficiency'' causing a lowering of blood pressure. An adjustment in steroid dose may be necessary.
- **Scanty, concentrated urine.** With dehydration, the kidneys try to conserve as much fluid as possible. The urine then becomes concentrated (dark yellow). If fluids cannot be taken by mouth because of associated nausea and vomiting, fluids may have to be provided by intravenous infusion.

If you experience any of these danger signals while traveling, consult a physician immediately.

There are occasional side effects to worry about, especially with doxycycline, which can cause rashes and increased sensitivity to the sun. Pediatric gastroenterologists may recommend a preventive dose of trimethoprim for their young patients when they travel into less developed countries, but here again, side effects must be considered.

If you do come down with traveler's diarrhea when on a trip, remember to drink plenty of fluids and take extra salt to prevent dehydration. Water or weak tea is perhaps preferable to citrus drinks or soda (both of which may increase motility and could accentuate the diarrhea). Lukewarm fluids are preferable to ice cold beverages, which also may increase diarrhea. Such standard antidiarrheal medications as Lomotil® and Imodium® relieve cramps and reduce general discomfort. Be sure to follow your doctor's instructions regarding these medications and their dosages to avoid any possibility of complications of your IBD that could be caused by overusage of these preparations. Remember that the illness is often short-lived, with more than half of patients improving within two days and three- quarters within four days.

Travel out of the U.S. also exposes us to different, more exotic foods and cooking preparations. Cruise ships and international hotel chains provide "international" cuisine which is much like standard American fare, but local restaurants and cafés may serve food which is much spicier or much oilier that what we are used to. If spices or greasy foods do not sit well in your stomach or intestines at home, they probably won't when you are on vacation. In tropical countries, there is an abundance of fruit available, so be certain not to overindulge in roughage which can cause looseness of the stool or aggravate an underlying bowel obstruction.

Some IBD sufferers may worry that the risk of travel to Latin America and other less developed countries are going to make them so anxious that their trip will be spoiled. In that case, consider a cruise to the Pacific Coast of Mexico or in the Caribbean. Hawaii, the Virgin Islands and Puerto Rico all provide a U.S.-style version of the tropics as do South Florida and the Florida Keys, with little worry about traveler's diarrhea.

Questions for Your Physician

Before any trip you will need certain answers from your physician:

1. "What if I have a mild flare-up when I'm away?" Have a written plan for increase in your medication dose and for the use of antispasmodic or antidiarrheal (Lomotil,® Imodium,® codeine, etc.) medications. What should you do about diet under these circumstances? Again, have a written plan of action regarding dietary modifications.

2. "What if I have a fairly serious flare-up when I'm away?" Obtain a written plan for taking prednisone or antibiotics under these circumstances (e.g. how much and for how many days and in what dosage). Have an adequate supply in case doses need to be raised.

3. "When should I consult a local physician (preferably a gastroenterologist)?" Find out from your physician which are the serious symptoms to look for, but don't ruin your trip by expecting a flare-up to occur.

4. "How about names of physicians who could help me?" Many physicians have colleagues overseas whom they know from their training days or from medical meetings and conferences. Some of them may live and practice in cities you will be visiting. Your doctor can find names and addresses of overseas members of American gastroenterological organizations who will have high levels of skill.

Finally, as you travel, be aware of people around you who could be of help should a medical problem arise. Befriend a physician on your trip and do not be embarrassed about asking for advice or help if the need arises. If a physician is not on your tour, there may be one staying at your hotel. Also bear in mind that other members of the health field, such as nurses, can also be extremely helpful.

Part V

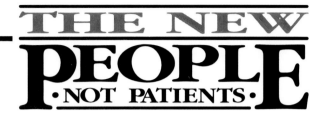

Knowing Your Rights

Paying for Your Health Care

20

In many ways, the health insurance picture in the U.S. is considerably bleaker now than it was in the mid-1980s when the first edition of this book was published. Since then, soaring health care costs and a worsening economy have caused many health insurance companies to be far more selective about whom they insure. Younger, healthier people frequently pay lower premiums than those who are older or have a "significant" medical history. Now in open competition with each other for the healthiest subscribers, many insurers deliberately offer employers skimpy benefit packages—such as low reimbursements for medications and hospitalizations—so as to discourage those with a need to use health services from enrolling in the plan. In a disturbing trend, some health insurers have begun to deny coverage to individuals engaged in certain professions—professional dancers, waiters, florists, etc.—in order to avoid enrolling anyone whom they think might be infected with the AIDS virus.

Employers hit by skyrocketing insurance premiums are reappraising how much they want to spend on their employees' health benefits or whether they will continue to offer health insurance at all.

As if this weren't enough, employers hit by skyrocketing insurance premiums are reappraising how much they want to spend on their employees' health benefits or whether they will continue to offer health insurance at all. Some employers change insurance carriers every few years, taking advantage of lower premiums but exposing workers in less-than-perfect health to the risk of being excluded altogether. Even worse, employees with chronic conditions have been singled out and told to limit health expenditures or look for other jobs; the message they are getting from employers is that their insurance premiums are costing the company too much. Taken together, these trends do not bode well for the person with IBD.

How Health Insurance Works

In the absence of a national program covering all Americans, health insurance in the U.S. is a patchwork quilt of coverage ranging from for-profit commercial insurers to Blue Cross plans to health maintenance organizations (HMOs) to government programs such as Medicare and Medicaid. Most Americans depend on the health insurance they (or family members) obtain at work through commercial carriers or Blue Cross/Blue Shield plans.

Far from attempting to screen out the sick, Blue Cross plans evolved in the post-depression years as a way to ensure that groups of people in a community, such as teachers, could pay their hospital bills, and that as many people as possible would be covered. Blue Cross became known for its policy of "community rating": everyone in a community, from workers in large corporations to individual policy holders, was considered part of the same "risk pool" and paid the same rates, sick or well.

HMOs: A Good Choice for the Person with IBD?

Under federal law, any company that offers health insurance plans and has at least 25 employees must give its workers the option to choose between a traditional health plan and an HMO. HMOs (health maintenance organizations) are for-profit health organizations that encourage subscribers to maintain their health through access to regular primary care, hospitalization when necessary, and the use of preventive health services. Rather than paying a fee for each service used (as in a traditional health plan), the subscriber—usually the employer—pays a set annual fee in monthly installments regardless of the number of services used, including hospitalization, thus eliminating most out-of-pocket expenses and paperwork. The range of services offered by HMOs is substantial and usually includes:

- physician visits
- in-patient and out-patient hosptial services in HMO affiliated hospitals
- diagnostic tests and x-rays
- emergency room services
- preventive health services, such as screening tests, etc.

If you think all this sounds too good to be true for the person with IBD, you may be right. To keep costs down and stay in business, the HMO must attract healthy working people who use fewer medical services; it must also try to keep members out of the hospital. If you join an HMO *before* you develop IBD, you will be fully covered. Unfortunately, joining an HMO *after* you have developed IBD may be much more difficult, since HMOs cover pre-existing conditions only if they are specifically written into a group policy.

A second way that HMOs control the use of services (and their costs) is to use primary care physicians (non-specialists) as "gatekeepers," who can then decide whether your episode of illness merits the use of one of the HMO's specialists. If you already have a professional relationship with a gastroenterologist of your choice who is not a member of the HMO, you will have to pay for physician visits yourself. Nevertheless, an undetermined number of people with IBD who can live with these restrictions obtain good health care through HMOs.

Blue Cross found itself covering sicker people and began to charge higher and higher premiums just to stay in business.

With increasing competition from commercial insurers who make their money by insuring as many healthy people as possible, Blue Cross found itself covering sicker people and began to charge higher and higher premiums just to stay in business. With prepaid health plans such as HMOs (see box) also attracting healthier employees, many Blue Cross plans that still insure those with "pre-existing conditions" have become *de facto* risk pools for the chronically ill. This is particularly true in states such as Minnesota, New Jersey, New York, and Pennsylvania, where Blue Cross/Blue Shield plans continue to enroll people with pre-existing conditions and offer generous, though expensive, benefit packages. Even so, Empire Blue Cross/Blue Shield of New York State recently dropped group coverage for 100,000 members of professional and trade associations—such as local chambers of commerce and journalist groups—claiming that it kept losing money on the "older and sicker" members of such groups.

Obtaining Health Insurance at Work

Because people with IBD and other chronic conditions *do* cost more for hospital and office care than people without these conditions, the person with IBD is considered a high risk to an insurer. Nevertheless, since most insurers offer group health benefits through employers, the liability of carrying a high-risk employee is spread over a larger group of healthy employees. This makes it possible, in most cases, for a working person with a pre-existing condition like IBD to obtain group coverage. Premiums for group coverage are usually paid by employers, although, increasingly, many companies are requiring co-payments from employees.

Fortunately, most people with Crohn's disease or ulcerative colitis are healthy enough to work at regular jobs, or are covered as dependents under the health insurance policy of a family member (See results of CCFA survey on the next page). But even if you can obtain health insurance at work, you may find that the policy offered by your employer does not cover pre-existing conditions until after a full year of employment, or will cover them only after a fixed period of time during which you are "symptom-free" or "treatment-free."

Obviously, if it is at all possible to choose, the person with IBD would do far better with a larger employer, at least as far as health insurance is concerned.

It is also true that the larger the company you work for, the more generous the medical coverage is likely to be and, in most cases, the fewer the restrictions in covering persons with chronic conditions. Conversely, a smaller company may offer a less comprehensive medical insurance policy with more restrictions, if they offer health insurance at all. A recent survey by the Health Insurance Association of America found that only a third of companies with fewer than 10 employees offered workers any health insurance. Obviously, if it is at all possible to choose, the person with IBD would do far better with a larger employer, at least as far as health insurance is concerned. In any case, be sure to ask about medical benefits *before* you are hired. (See Chapter 21 for a discussion of your rights to health insurance access on the job under the new Americans with Disabilities Act of 1990.)

What Kind of Health Plan Should I Have?

A good health insurance plan for the person with IBD should offer the maximum number of hospital days (usually 120 or 365) per year in a semi-private room. (A much poorer choice is a plan offering to pay a flat amount per hospital day, a so-called hospital indemnity plan.) The major-medical portion of your plan should cover physician services in the hospital, as well as diagnostic and laboratory procedures such as endoscopy, x-rays and other tests. Most plans pay after the first $200, $500 or more deductible (your out-of-pocket expenses), and then only up to a certain percentage, usually 80 percent, of your total charges. Some plans require co-payments for physician charges.

Coverage for office visits to your physician is also very important. Unfortunately, many plans do not pay for these unless they are "diagnosis-related." This is fine for your IBD visits to your gastroenterologist or surgeon, but not for regular primary or preventive care.

In an effort to contain costs, many insurers now enforce "managed care" programs, requiring policy holders to obtain prior approval or a second opinion before entering the hospital or having surgery. Others use a list of "preferred providers"; using a physician not on the list may mean that you will pay half of the bill yourself.

Changing or Losing a Job: What Happens to Your Health Insurance?

Today, many people—and not just those with chronic illnesses—are reluctant to change jobs because of the uncertainty about whether they will obtain any health

CCFA Health Insurance Survey Results: Less-than-Adequate Coverage and Anxiety about the Future

A recent national survey of members of voluntary health agencies, including the CCFA, asked a sample of Americans with chronic disabling conditions what kind of health insurance they had and how adequately that insurance met their needs. Fifty-eight people with IBD responded to the survey, not enough to draw any definitive conclusions for IBD sufferers as a whole, but certainly enough to draw attention to the health insurance problems we face.

Overall, 93 percent of the respondents with IBD had some kind of private health insurance: most (83 percent) were insured as part of a group plan through their (or a spouse's) employer; 17 percent had individual plans. About half had Blue Cross/Blue Shield coverage, a third had commercial insurance carriers, and the remaining 19 percent had joined an HMO.

While these numbers sound reassuring, they conceal some basic problems in the breadth of health insurance coverage for conditions like IBD. Although 64 percent of respondents reported having full coverage for hospital care (27 percent had partial coverage), only 48 percent were fully covered for physician services, and 16 percent had no coverage at all for these services. HMO members did better than Blue Cross or commercial subscribers in both these areas. What is more, 30 percent of the responding CCFA members said their current insurance policies *excluded* coverage of IBD, making people with IBD one of the more vulnerable patient groups subject to exclusion by pre-existing condition. One third reported being rejected for health insurance in the past because of IBD, and another one third reported spending more than 10 percent of the family income for out-of-pocket health expenses in the last year.

(Continued on next page)

coverage for themselves or their dependents in a new job. For those with a positive medical history or with illness in a family member, health insurance can trap them in jobs or even in careers they no longer want. Some of these workers even avoid using their insurance unless absolutely necessary, fearing that the policy may be cancelled.

For those with a positive medical history or with illness in a family member, health insurance can trap them in jobs or even in careers they no longer want.

Losing a job is another reason to be concerned about the loss of health insurance. Depending on what state you live in and the type of group policy offered in your former company, you may be able to convert to individual or family health coverage. Nevertheless, an individual health insurance plan will cost you much more than you would have spent for group coverage (since you become a risk pool of one!) and benefits will be fewer. For example, if your group health plan at work offered major-medical benefits (hospital, out-patient doctor visits, and laboratory tests, etc.), the conversion policy offered to you by the insurer may offer only hospital benefits and reimbursements for in-hospital physician visits. The high cost of such plans reflects the fact that most people who buy this type of coverage are in poor health, since insurers may not deny conversion because of ill health.

The following 15 states **do not** require employers to offer conversion policies to employees who leave: Alabama, Alaska, Connecticut, Delaware, Hawaii, Idaho, Indiana, Louisiana, Massachusetts, Michigan, Mississippi, Nebraska, New Jersey, North Dakota, and Oklahoma.

COBRA: What Is It and How Can It Help You?

To remedy the large-scale problem of loss of health insurance caused by job loss, Congress passed the Consolidated Omnibus Budget Reconciliation Act of 1985, or COBRA. COBRA allows workers leaving companies with 20 or more employees to continue medical coverage for 18 months under a former employers's group plan, and up to 36 months if health insurance was lost through divorce or the death of a covered spouse. You must pay the full cost of your premium plus a 2 percent administrative charge. Nevertheless, insurance advocates agree that for the short term, COBRA is a better deal, both in premium cost and breadth of coverage, than conversion to an individual plan. By law, after your employer notifies you of your COBRA rights, you have 60 days to begin paying premiums or refuse coverage. Once you decline benefits under COBRA, you will no longer be eligible for them. Because pre-existing conditions are covered under COBRA (if they were covered under your group plan), you can continue under COBRA for the balance of the 18 months, even if the health plan on your new job has a waiting period.

Risk Pools: Insurers of Last Resort

Health insurance risk pools were created to provide medical coverage for the approximately one million Americans who have been denied commercial health insurance because of chronic illness. These plans offer both individual and family coverage and they cannot discriminate against a person because of income. There are two major drawbacks: the cost can be very high and risk pools are operative in only a few states. Although legislation has

(Continued from previous page)

Most of the 19 percent of respondents covered by HMOs were very pleased with their medical coverage and relieved of worries about hospital and doctor bills. Others, however, expressed concerns about changing jobs, fearful that they would be unable to duplicate their HMO coverage elsewhere. Said one Michigan man, "I'm stuck in a job I don't particularly like with a limited future. I think I would have left years ago if not for the worries about medical insurance."

Those with Blue Cross or commercial health insurance seemed fairly satisfied and even grateful to have any insurance at all. However, some reported having policies with huge deductibles—up to $2,000 or even $5,000—, large out-of-pocket expenses, and no coverage for ostomy supplies. Some of those with Crohn's disease said they lived in fear of using up the lifetime maximum benefits on their policies because of the need for costly total parenteral nutrition (TPN) treatments. Others worried that their employers might go bankrupt, leaving them to fend for themselves in an insurance market they feel is stacked against them.

The Vulnerable Uninsured: 18 to 24 Year-Olds

Of all age groups lacking health insurance, by far the largest is young adults aged 18 to 24. Much too young for Medicare and usually ineligible for Medicaid because of requirements that they have children, young adults make up 25 percent of the estimated 37 million uninsured Americans. It's not difficult to understand why this is so.

Covered while they are students, many young people "age-out" of their parents' health plans when they leave high school or college. Unless they find work right away, they may go for long periods of time without health insurance. A recent survey of the health insurance status of young adults found that unemployment—coupled with the high cost of coverage—was the reason why most 18 to 24 year-olds lacked health insurance. Hardest hit are young people who are less educated, poor, and live in rural areas.

Even when they do find work, young adults tend to hold down part-time, temporary, or lower-paying jobs, jobs that usually offer no health benefits. Although they are healthier than most older workers, they may not be employed by companies large enough to offer them coverage through an HMO. Of course, many 18 to 24 year-olds don't anticipate getting sick and may not even think they need health insurance.

This is certainly not the case for young adults with IBD, who are painfully aware of the importance of health insurance. Perhaps the most important thing a parent can do for a son or daughter with IBD is to plan for continuation of medical coverage—if at all possible—*before* the upper age limit is reached. The reason this is so important is because many Blue Cross and commercial carriers will not enforce restrictions on pre-existing conditions if coverage with them has been continuous. If health insurance is allowed to lapse, it may be difficult or impossible for your son or daughter to obtain coverage again—working or not.

been passed mandating the establishment of risk pools in 23 states, pools are now operating in only the following 16 states: Connecticut, Florida, Illinois, Indiana, Iowa, Maine, Minnesota, Montana, Nebraska, New Mexico, North Dakota, Oregon, South Carolina, Tennessee, Washington, and Wisconsin. Work is still underway to put plans into effect in California, Colorado, Georgia, Louisiana, Texas, Utah, and Wyoming, resulting in waiting lists of up to a year for the scarce policies.

Once legislation establishing a risk pool is signed into law in a state, all the health insurance firms within that state form an association. One firm is then selected to administer a plan from which eligible state residents can purchase health insurance. Some states require that an applicant show proof of ineligibility for Medicare or Medicaid coverage, or proof of rejection by a commercial carrier. Three states (Illinois, Maine, and Oregon) limit the number of policies that can be issued.

State risk pools are far from the ideal solution to a problem that won't go away.

Nevertheless, compared with many commercial insurance policies, the coverage under a risk pool can be excellent. Many plans include physicians' fees, hospital services, home health care, prescription drugs, and skilled nursing care. Deductibles can be high, as much as $2,000 in some states, and premiums, set by the state insurance department are often exorbitant. Lifetime-benefit maximums are considerably lower than those offered under many Blue Cross/Blue Shield or commercial plans—$500,000 or even $250,000.

Although welcomed by those with nowhere else to turn for health insurance, state risk pools are far from the ideal solution to a problem that won't go away. They are a losing proposition for a state and must be funded by outside sources in order to survive. The insurance companies that underwrite these pools receive substantial tax breaks in exchange for their participation.

Summary

This chapter has offered some individual solutions to the worsening problem of obtaining health insurance to pay for the cost of treating IBD. Many people with IBD will be able to take advantage of one of the avenues to health insurance covered in this chapter. Others will be forced to join the ranks of the estimated 37 million Americans without any health insurance. Although a system of national health insurance for all Americans will not solve all the problems of access to proper health care, its eventual enactment will at least remove the major barrier to coverage encountered by those with chronic illnesses.

For further reading: You may write for a reprint of the excellent two-part article, entitled "The Crisis in Health Insurance," published by *Consumer Reports* in August and September, 1990. Write to:

Consumer Reports Reprints
P.O. Box CS 2010–A
Mount Vernon, NY 10551

Another helpful resource is the following:

Health Maintenance Organizations: What They Are, How They Work, and Which One Is Best for You by Jill Bloom. Published in paperback by The Body Press, Tuscon, AZ.

Dealing with Discrimination on the Job and at School

21

Most people with IBD don't want to think of themselves as disabled. The word "disabled" suggests a person who is confined to a wheel chair, or someone who is blind or has lost a limb. Yet, when Crohn's disease or ulcerative colitis limit our ability to attend school or report to work regularly, both illnesses can sometimes become handicapping conditions. Thinking in terms of disability is useful because it makes us familiar with laws that have been enacted to protect the disabled, and makes us aware of how these same laws might also protect the person with IBD.

Gains for the Disabled

Fortunately, Americans with many different kinds of disabling conditions—the physically and emotionally handicapped as well as the chronically ill—have benefitted greatly from protective laws passed during the 1970's, rightly called the "decade of disability." Thanks to lobbying efforts, demonstrations, protest marches and sit-ins by disability rights groups—tactics learned from the civil rights movement a decade earlier—Congress passed the 1973 Rehabilitation Act (Public Law 93–112). Section 504 of this law deals with non-discrimination under federal grants and reads:

"No otherwise qualified handicapped individual in the United States shall, on the basis of his/her handicap, be excluded from participation in, be denied the benefits of, or be subjected to discrimination under any program or activity receiving federal financial assistance."

This act was the single most powerful civil rights protection for the disabled ever enacted into law in this country. Section 504 prevents employers receiving federal monies (or those doing at least $2,500 in business with the federal government under Section 503) from refusing to hire the disabled, if reasonable accommodations can be made, and if the disability does not impair the performance of the job. It also means that such employers may not require pre-employment physical examinations. Any questions about disability are barred until an individual has been hired. The sweeping language of Section 504 also offers protection to the disabled in the public schools, in higher education, and in virtually all segments of American life which benefit from federal assistance. (The effects of Section 504 on education will be discussed later in this chapter.)

On July 26, 1990, Congress took an historic step to ensure the equal treatment of disabled people in virtually all areas of business, including private industry.

The Americans with Disabilities Act

The problem with the 1973 Rehabilitation Act was that employees of privately-owned buinesses, many state and local governments, and businesses that were not

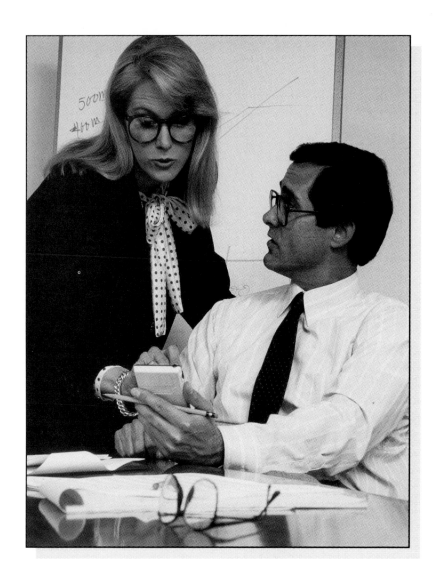

federal contractors were not covered. This left the majority of disabled or physically impaired Americans vulnerable to job loss because of a disability. On July 26, 1990, Congress took an historic step to ensure the equal treatment of disabled people in virtually all areas of business, including private industry. The Americans with Disabilities Act of 1990 (ADA), which will go into effect over the course of the next few years, will offer protection to disabled people against discrimination in all types of employment decisions, as well as in public accommodations, state and local government, and telecommunications.

The ADA broadly defines a disability as a "physical or mental impairment that substantially limits one or more of the major life activities." The ADA also states that anyone impaired by a "physiological disorder or condition" of the digestive system is considered disabled. Therefore, workers who have Crohn's disease or ulcerative colitis are protected by this act.

Your Rights as an Employee

On July 26, 1992, the employment provision of the ADA will take effect for firms that have 25 or more employees. By July 26, 1994, smaller businesses with 15 or more employees also will be bound by these guidelines.

The ADA protects "qualified" job applicants and employees who are disabled against discrimination in areas such as selection criteria, qualifications, and promotions. Thus, an employer cannot refuse to hire an applicant simply because that person has IBD. A disabled candidate is "qualified" if he/she can perform the fundamental tasks and responsibilities of a job, with "reasonable accommodation."

Accommodations are considered "unreasonable" if they cause an employer "undue hardship"—vaguely defined as

"significant difficulty or expense."
Unfortunately, the ADA provides no fixed
equations for calculating "significant
difficulty or expense." The interpretation
of "undue hardship" undoubtedly will be
established as courts throughout the country
consider individual discrimination cases.

Other ADA guidelines are clear. As they
are under the 1973 Rehabilitation Act,
inquiries about a job applicant's disability
are prohibited unless these questions have
a direct bearing on job performance. An
employer cannot ask a disabled person to
undergo a medical exam until he has offered
a job to that person. Information collected
from medical exams must be kept
confidential. A disabled person can be
denied a job *only* if an exam indicates that
he cannot perform the essential functions
of a job, even after reasonable
accommodations have been made.

ADA regulations mandate that
qualifications used to hire and to promote
disabled employees be job-related. For
example, an employer cannot deny a job to
an applicant because a family member has
IBD. (This may discourage employers from
discriminating against applicants whose
families may represent a high health
insurance expense.) Pre-employment tests
are acceptable only if they measure a potential
employee's ability to perform the essential
functions of a job (e.g., a typing test).

*Under ADA it would be illegal
for a company to refuse
to insure an employee
who has Crohn's disease,
while providing health benefits
for all other employees.*

Dos and Don'ts for the Working Person with IBD

- Keep the best work record possible. Remember that your employer pays your health insurance premiums as well as your salary.
- If any sick days are necessary, make sure they are documented by a physician's note, not just a "no show."
- Don't use your sick days for vacation. You may need them later in the year.
- Keep your illness to yourself. The job is not the place to impress fellow workers and your supervisor with how sick you can be.
- Try to look well no matter *how* you feel.
- Use your break time and meal time wisely— for healthy meals.
- Be honest with your supervisor and boss. If you get sick, warn them and give probable dates of return to work. This will allow them to plan for your absence.
- Use your health care benefits wisely so that your job and your benefits will be there when you need them.

Needed: A "Safety Net" for Workers with Sick Children

A Minnesota woman lost her job as an accounting clerk last year because she took off too many days from work to care for her sick child. What is worse, because she was fired for "misconduct," the state refused to pay her any unemployment benefits. The woman said she had no choice: "I had a sick baby and no one else to take care of him. I couldn't just leave him."

This kind of nightmare worries parents who must juggle the demands of jobs—usually for both parents—and the needs of a son or daughter with IBD. Many such parents speak privately of coming to work when they are ill and saving sick days in case they need to stay home with a sick youngster. This practice engenders guilt in the parents and may arouse suspicion—or even the envy—of fellow workers.

What's needed to remedy this dilemma experienced by *all* working parents—and especially those with a chronically ill child at home—is a federal family leave law that would protect parents' jobs while they take time off to care for sick children. Recognizing this need, Minnesota recently passed the nation's first law allowing parents to use some of their own sick leave to take care of an ill child. Just a few states—Connecticut, Maine, New Jersey, Rhode Island, Wisconsin, and the District of Columbia—have laws requiring employers to grant unpaid leave to workers with sick children. Other states extend this leave to state employees but not to those working for private companies. Unfortunately, last year President Bush vetoed a bill passed by both houses of Congress that would have provided a family leave for all workers requiring time off for family illness.

At this writing, Congress is considering another federal family leave bill. Passage—and Presidential endorsement—of such a bill would stop the practice of penalizing families with illnesses like IBD for trying to be good parents.

Employee Benefits under ADA

The ADA requires that employers provide identical insurance coverage to all employees. For example, under ADA it would be illegal for a company to refuse to insure an employee who has Crohn's disease, while providing health benefits for all other employees. However, the act does not require employers to anticipate the special needs of disabled employees. For example, an employer is not guilty of discrimination if the company's basic coverage does not provide reimbursement for total parental nutrition (TPN), a liquid nutritional formula that is administered intravenously. Moreover, the ADA allows employers to maintain benefit plans that do not provide coverage for pre-existing conditions.

On the other hand, an employer cannot limit coverage *after* experience with a disabled employee. For instance, the ADA prohibits employers from lowering the cap on TPN costs after reviewing the high expense incurred by an employee. Neither can a company offer a benefit cap of $10,000 to employees who have IBD, while all other employees receive maximum coverage of $100,000.

Your Rights in Other Areas

The ADA stipulates that bathrooms in "public accommodations" (bars, restaurants, schools, etc.) must be accessible to people who have disabilities. However, public accommodations are still free to establish their own policies concerning the use of their restrooms. For example, a restaurant may maintain a "patrons only" policy and prohibit a passerby who has IBD from using its restroom.

It is critical that people who have IBD understand fully their rights under this landmark legislation. Though some of the ADA's provisions and terms will have to be clarified either through additional legislation or through litigation, the Americans with Disabilities Act of 1990 represents a substantial breakthrough for everyone who is affected by IBD. **For more information, call the United States Department of Justice ADA Hotline at (202) 514–0301.**

Education for the Disabled

The 1973 Rehabilitation Act has also paved the way for full access to education for children with physical, emotional or medical impairments. In 1975, Congress passed the Education for All Handicapped Children Act (Public Law 94–142), requiring a free, public education for all children with a disability. The law contains strong incentives for the states to comply, namely the threatened loss of millions of federal dollars in aid to education. In addition, this legislation has created a climate in the schools where non-disabled students and teachers will gain an understanding of what it means to be disabled through increased exposure to students who are "mainstreamed" into their schools.

For the student with IBD, this means that there is increased leverage for the accessibility of school bathrooms, and that the public school must provide home or in-hospital instruction at no cost to the parents when a child with IBD is too ill to attend school. While these laws will not erase overnight the insensitivity to physical and medical disability found in so many schools, they should give students and their parents the confidence to press for what are now their clear legal rights.

It is still important for the student and his/her parents to assist teachers and school personnel in understanding how best to address the particular problems IBD poses for the student. CCFA's brochure,

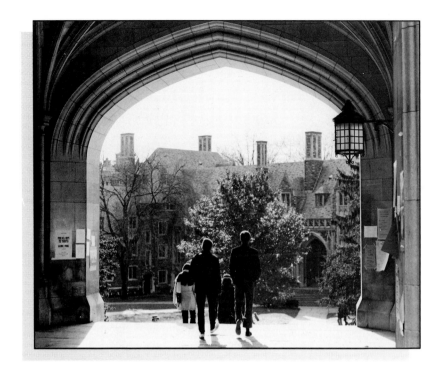

"A Teacher's Guide to Crohn's Disease and Ulcerative Colitis," was specifically developed to accomplish this purpose.

Access to Higher Education

Section 504 and the Education of All Handicapped Children Act broke new ground in higher education as well, assuring non-discrimination in admissions, placement, housing, financial aid, and in all aspects of student life at colleges and universities. Under Section 504, college and university publications, brochures, and applications must contain a statement of non-discrimination on the basis of handicap in the recruitment and admission of students. Inquiry about a physical or medical impairment may be made only *after* admission of a student. Medical information can be solicited, for example through a medical examination, after an applicant has been admitted if the medical information obtained is not used for the purpose of excluding or disqualifying anyone who is qualified to participate in any of the institution's programs or activities.

The student with IBD who is applying to college should remember that under Section 504, he/she is *not required* to reveal any information about the facts or history of his/her illness. This applies as well to those persons sending letters of recommendation in the student's behalf. However, under certain circumstances, it may be advantageous for the student to disclose the fact of his/her illness, for example when high school grades have suffered because of time spent in the hospital. A letter from the student's physician stating the facts should alert the admissions office to the reasons for long absences from school and the potential medical needs of the student while on campus. However, under Section 504, it is the responsibility of the interviewer or admissions officer *not* to use this information about the student's medical impairment to influence decisions about admissions.

Section 504 also requires that student orientation programs must be accessible to all students. Some colleges and universities have adopted the practice of holding week-long orientation sessions for freshmen in a camp setting where there is little or no access to toilet facilities. Needless to say, this type of situation presents enormous problems for the students with IBD, who may choose to avoid the orientation altogether. College officials may need some further prompting from parents as to what constitutes an impediment to full participation in college life. Again, the student with IBD and his/her family must take the lead.

If you feel that you have been denied admission to a college or university or have not been permitted to participate fully in campus life on the basis of your handicap (medical impairment), you or your authorized representative should file a written complaint with the college or university. The complaint should explain:

- Who was discriminated against.
- In what way.
- By whom of which institution.
- When the discrimination took place.
- Who was harmed by the discriminatory act.
- Who can be contacted for the information.
- Your name, address, zip code and telephone number.
- As much background information as possible.

If you are not satisfied with the response you get, file a written complaint with the Office for Civil Rights, Department of Health and Human Services, Washington D.C., 20201.

Obtaining and Understanding Your Medical Records

22

Anyone familiar with the rise of consumerism in the health field would argue that the appetite of the American public for medical information is increasing dramatically. Consumer groups are compiling physician directories and pushing for increased health awareness among all sectors of the population. A glance at the health book section in any book store reveals a flood of new titles on every aspect of health and disease. This new awareness also takes the form of an intense desire for control over information about the health care we are receiving and paying for. Yet the one document which is likely to contain the greatest amount of information pertinent to our personal health—the medical record—often remains inaccessible. This chapter will explain what is contained in the medical record, why it is important for the person with IBD to have access to that record (or to parts of it), and how to go about obtaining it.

What Is in Your Hospital Medical Record?

Your hospital medical record contains documentation about why you were admitted to the hospital, what laboratory tests and diagnostic procedures were performed while you were there, what were the results, and what was your progress (or lack of it) during the hospital stay. This record is both a valuable communication tool between the members of the health care team who care for you and an important legal document of the care you have received while in the hospital. Your record begins to accumulate

forms from the moment you enter the admitting office and are assigned a unit number; information is added to your record until, and even after, you leave the hospital. The "chart," as it is called by hospital personnel, is kept at the nurses' station on your unit, and all hospital personnel who participate in your care are required to make entries regarding your treatment. After you are discharged, your record is sent to the medical record department of the hospital. When all forms are completed and signed, your record is then filed under the number assigned to you at admission. Subsequent hospital admissions will use this same unit number, so that information on multiple hospitalizations is bound together in one record.

Users of the Medical Record

The medical record is legally the property of the hospital, and whether or not you have the right to see or have a copy of your medical record depends on what laws have been passed in your state. At the same time, the *information* contained in the record is confidential in nature and is "owned" by the patient. For this reason, anyone admitted to a hospital must sign a release authorizing the hospital to permit inspection of the record by insurance companies, Blue Cross, or government payers (Medicare, Medicaid) in order to verify the care that has been rendered. In addition, the broad wording of most release-of-information authorizations permits access to your record by law enforcement agencies, schools, social

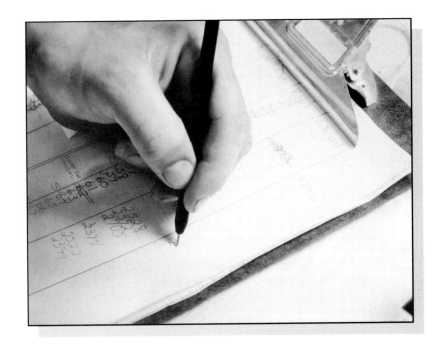

service agencies, hospital risk managers, and by medical researchers on the hospital staff. Moreover, insurance companies pool the information obtained from claims review in a large computerized data bank of which most people are totally unaware. Hospital patients have asked, logically, how they can possibly make an informed decision to authorize the use of their records by third parties when they themselves have not seen those records and have no idea what they contain.

The Importance of Access

In these days of increased participation by people in their own health care, the arguments favoring patient access to the medical record are stronger than ever. This is especially true for persons with a chronic illness such as IBD. In the past, members of the medical profession have sought to prevent patient access to this information, claiming that patients could not possibly understand their charts. Unfortunately, some doctors interpret these requests from their patients as a loss of trust rather than as a desire to learn more about their conditions. Recently, however, the American Hospital Association, in a reversal of its earlier position, has taken a stand on supporting the right of patients to obtain complete medical information from doctors, provided they will not be harmed medically by what they read.

Access to pertinent medical record information means that "patients" can start acting more like "consumers" in selecting the best health care available to them and avoiding unnecessary and costly procedures.

People have little to lose and a lot to gain from seeing all or part of their hospital records. First, there is the obvious sense of relief at having the secrecy removed from the record, together with the more open physician-patient partnership which is likely to result. Access to written records also increases a person's sense of responsibility in making important health care decisions. Possession of at least a part of the record, such as the Discharge Summary, Operative Report, Endoscopy Report, Pathology Report, and the results and actual copies of recent x-rays, is helpful in assuring continuity of care when a person changes physicians, moves to another part of the country, or is in an emergency situation requiring immediate access to medical information. Access to pertinent medical record information means that "patients" can start acting more like "consumers" in selecting the best health care available to them and avoiding unnecessary and costly procedures.

Gaining Access to Your Records

Whether or not you have legal access to your hospital records depends upon where you live. Since the hospital is the legal owner of the record, right to access can be granted only by state laws (statutes) or by case law in a particular state. State laws vary greatly as to the types of records covered (i.e. hospital records or doctor's office records), who has access to those records (i.e. patient, attorney or physician), and the form of access (i.e. whether a patient is entitled to see or copy the record, or is entitled to a summary only.)

A number of states now provide for some sort of patient access (direct or indirect) to both hospital and doctor's records. Several states grant access to hospital records only. This leaves about half the states with no statutes at all.

The Parts of Your Hospital Record

The following forms are standard parts of all hospital medical records:

face sheet—contains admitting and billing information (name, address, employer, insurance carrier), admitting diagnosis. Final diagnosis is added upon discharge.

admission note—records your condition on admission, including results of recent tests.

history and physical examination—contains your complete medical history as told to the admitting resident, as well as results of physical examination.

graphic record—a record of your temperature, pulse, respiration and blood pressure while in the hospital.

progress notes—a daily record of your progress, test results, etc. by the professionals who care for you.

doctor's order sheets—a record of the medications ordered for you by your physicians.

x-ray reports—results of diagnostic x-rays.

laboratory reports—results of various tests.

nursing notes, admitting forms and medication record—separate entries made by the nursing staff.

operative report—a complete record of any operation dictated by the surgeon after surgery.

pathology report—results of examination of any tissues removed from your body at operation or biopsy.

discharge summary—a summary dictated by your physician during or after the hospital stay, including any tests or operations performed, laboratory data, your condition on discharge, and plans for your follow-up care.

To check on your right to access in your state, you should write or call the Public Citizen Health Research Group, 2000 P Street, N.W., Washington, D.C. 20036. To find out if there are any medical record access bills pending in your state, write to your state assemblyman or state senator.

The following steps are recommended by the Public Citizen Health Research Group for individuals interested in obtaining their health records:

1. **Check the statutes in your state**—Even if your state is one of those having no statute granting access, the states generally have no statutes *denying* access, and hospitals or doctors are always free to grant access if they wish.

2. **Contact the hospital or doctor**—Ask what procedure you should follow, e.g. going in person to the hospital's medical record department or putting your request in writing. If you are refused access, cite the applicable law in your state and make notes of the response.

3. **Submit a written request**—If you have been unsuccessful in obtaining your record, cite the relevant law in your letter and be specific about the part or parts of the record you wish to obtain. (Consult the chart at the beginning of this chapter; the most useful documents to you are likely to be the Discharge Summary, Operative Report and X-Ray Reports.) The hospital may charge you a fee for these copies. Keep a copy of your correspondence.

What to Do if Your Request Is Denied

If you live in a state where there is no statute permitting access to medical records and if your request to a provider has been denied, you may consider using the help of patient rights groups in your area. However, the most successful way around this obstacle is to have the hospital release a copy of your record to a physician who will share the information with you. Since you are the "owner" of the information contained in the record, you must be the one to authorize this release. Even this may be unnecessary, since the physician who took care of you in the hospital usually keeps copies of your Discharge Summary, Operative Report and X-Ray Reports with the office records, and will often share these with you even if not required to do so by law. Failing this, you may wish to have your lawyer make a request for your records in your behalf. The last resort, of course, is to sue the health care provider. The other course of action is to work toward passage of an access bill in your state.

Access to Records in Federal Facilities

Under the Privacy Act of 1974, patients in Veteran's Administration hospitals, Public Health Service hospitals, or military hospitals have the right to inspect, copy, and correct information in their medical records. You should first telephone the hospital to determine the procedures you should follow. You may be required to submit a written request. If for any reason you are unable to obtain these records, you should write to:

Freedom of Information Clearinghouse
P.O. Box 19367
Washington, D.C. 20036

Obtaining Copies of Your X-Rays

X-rays performed in the hospital or physician's office are a valuable record of the course of your IBD. They are often required for comparison over the years of illness and treatment. Hospitals and physicians are required by law to keep x-rays for a period of time (as defined by state law). After this time period, x-rays are either destroyed or sold to retrieve the silver content of the film itself. Before they are destroyed, or at any time, you may request that a copy be made (at your expense). Many physicians will simply give these older x-rays to their patients as a record of treatment. Together with the written hospital or office record, x-rays enable a person with IBD to have a basic understanding of the course of IBD treatment.

Understanding Your Records

The medical record contains many words and abbreviations which you may not understand at first. This medical terminology, medical jargon, or "medicalese," as it is often called, is a kind of universal convenient shorthand used by physicians, nurses, and all other health care workers to communicate quickly about the patients they care for. While you can easily look up any terms or words you don't understand in any good medical dictionary, you may have more trouble deciphering the abbreviations you will encounter.

Listed here are some of the most common abbreviations and the parts of the chart where they are likely to appear.

History and Physical Examination

ABD—abdomen
CC—chief complaint
CD—Crohn's disease
Dx—diagnosis
EENT—eye, ear, nose, and throat
BP—blood pressure
BM—bowel movements
GB—gallbladder
GI—gastrointestinal
HEENT—head, eyes, ears, nose and throat
H & L—heart and lungs
H & P or HPE—history and/or physical examination
Hx—history
KLS—kidney, liver and spleen
LLQ—left lower quadrant (of abdomen)
LUQ—left upper quadrant (of abdomen)
NAD—no apparent distress
NSR—normal sinus rhythm (of the heart)
O—eye
O2—both eyes
P & A—percussion and auscultation (techniques for examinating the abdomen and thorax)
Palp—palpation (of organs in the abdomen)
RLQ—right lower quadrant
RUQ—right upper quadrant
Rx—medications
SB—small bowel
TPR—temperature, pulse and respiration
Tx—treatment
UC—ulcerative colitis
WNL—within normal limits
VS—vital signs
WD/WN—well-developed and well-nourished

Laboratory and Diagnostic Tests

Alb—albumin
BE—barium enema
Cath—catheter
CBC—complete blood count
C & S—culture and sensitivity (tests for bacteria in blood and urine samples)
CX—chest x-ray
ECG—electrocardiogram
EN—enema
ESR—erythrocyte sedimentation rate
Ex—examination
Fx—fluoroscopy
Hb, Hgb—hemoglobin
Hct—hematocrit
IVP—intravenous pyelogram
RBC—red blood cell
SMA-12—automated test of blood chemistries
TIBC—total iron binding capacity
UGIS—upper gastrointestinal series
US—ultrasound
WBC—white blood cell

Physicians' and Nurses' Orders

(many of these abbreviations stem from Latin terms)

AC—before meals (*ante cibum*)
BID—twice a day (*bis in die*)
c̄—with (*cum*)
HS—hour of sleep (*hora somni*)
IM—intramuscular
IV—intravenous
NPO—nothing by mouth (*nihil per os*)
PC—after meals (*post cibum*)
PO—by mouth (*per os*)
PRN—as needed (*pro re nata*)
QD—every day
q4h—every four hours
QOD—every other day
R/O—rule out
s̄—without
SOS—when necessary (*si opus sit*)
STAT—immediately
TID—three times a day

For Further Information

Annas, George J., *The Rights of Hospital Patients*. New York: Avon Books, 1975.

Sarath, Maria, Auerbach, Melissa, and Bogue, Ted. *Medical Records: Getting Yours*. Washington, D.C.: Public Citizen Health Research Group, 1980.

Afterword

The Last 50 Years in IBD: A Long and Winding Trail

This epilogue to a book devoted to the person with IBD will survey what we have all learned along the way in this long winding trail toward the ultimate discovery of cause and cure.

A useful way to see how far we have come despite the gaps in our knowledge about IBD is to look at where we were 50 or so years ago. Join me, therefore, as an anxious intern going out on wards of the Mt. Sinai Hospital in 1939. How could we study and diagnose IBD then and what did we have to treat these patients? We depended a great deal on the history of symptoms, examined the stool for blood and pus, looked into the rectum with a rigid sigmoidoscope, and sent the stool off to the laboratory to be sure we had not overlooked a parasite or specific "bug." We had available to us x-rays to do a barium enema and we would take pictures of the remainder of the gut by giving barium by mouth and tediously following its course throughout the small bowel. Although we have learned new endoscopic and radiographic techniques, these were not too different from what we use nowadays.

If patients and family are disappointed in our slow progress toward cure of their illnesses— and doctors and researchers are frustrated—consider how far we have come in this arduous search.

But how did we treat our patients in 1939? Not very well and not with many medicines. For ulcerative colitis we would give intravenous fluid, some sugar water, and electrolytes, but we had no way of improving nutrition with intravenous calories, proteins and fats. There was no possibility of giving IV feedings at home. We treated anemia with blood transfusions; indeed we had so little to offer patients, even if they were not anemic, that we gave them transfusions, little ones daily, just to pick them up. No worry about AIDS in 1939! If the patient were very sick with ulcerative colitis, we would try to put the bowel at rest by doing an ileostomy, but it didn't seem to work. We were also more daring in very toxic patients by taking out the whole colon; this was risky since we had no antibiotics except sulfanilamide to fight infections and our ileostomies were difficult to manage.

For "regional ileitis," the only form of Crohn's disease we knew of, we were happy to make the the diagnosis and tell the patient that the cause of his or her suffering was in the small intestine and not in the head! As for medical treatment, we could do nothing except to recommend removal of the areas of the small intestine that were involved. This we did in stages, the first being a bypass of the inflamed area. Some patients felt so much better that we often skipped the second stage of removing the bypassed part, which we have come to regret. Now we make every effort to remove badly diseased bowel in order to prevent a cancer developing in the bypassed loop of intestine.

Such was the dismal situation just a half century ago. If patients and family are disappointed in our slow progress toward cure of their illnesses—and doctors and researchers *are* frustrated—consider how far we have come in this arduous search. In ulcerative colitis, we can suppress mild and moderately active disease with corticosteroids, sulfasalazine, and 5-ASA medications and even induce longer remissions. If all else fails, we can cure the disease by removing the colon at the price of an ileostomy. But today's ileostomy is much improved and we now have the option of newer operations that do not require external appliances.

In Crohn's disease, we can improve the patient's lot with sulfasalazine, steroids, antibiotics, and immunosuppressive agents. We can treat the complications of stricture, abscess and fistula surgically by removing minimal amounts of bowel or performing strictureplasty.

For both diseases, we can vastly improve nutritional status with enteral or parental means and continue nutritional support at home. Complete recovery from an operation for Crohn's disease or ulcerative colitis is now the rule and not the exception.

Each advance in the diagnosis and management of IBD was hard-won and took time and concerted effort by scores of researchers, clinicians and laboratories. There are no short cuts. Discoveries in IBD, as in all of medicine, depend on both skill and chance, and take time. We have really known about IBD for a little more than 50 years of the modern era in medicine. So with our patients we grab at straws, hope for short cuts, and are influenced by fashion. For example there are fashions in diet that come and go. Lactose intolerance is not synonymous with IBD and removal of milk and milk products does not always help. The nutritional problems of our patients have called forth a huge cry for nutritional cures, but megavitamins and bizarre diets have led only to disappointment. Acupuncture has had its day. Naturopaths and coffee enemas have lured the unwary.

If something is hidden, the way to find it, I believe, is to have lots of people look for it in a lot of places. Since the founding of the National Foundation for Ileitis and Colitis, now fittingly called the Crohn's and Colitis Foundation of America, a lot of smart researchers are out looking for solutions to our problems in all sorts of places. It is always dangerous to predict when answers will be found, but when they are found they may turn out to be simple.

Henry D. Janowitz, M.D.
Chairman Emeritus
National Scientific Advisory Committee

Appendix A

Educational Resources for People with IBD Published by the Crohn's & Colitis Foundation of America, Inc.

Brochures:

Questions and Answers about Crohn's
   Disease and Ulcerative Colitis

Preguntas y Repuestas acerca de la
   Enfermedad Crohn y Colitis Ulcerativa
   (Spanish version of above brochure)

Questions and Answers about Diet and
   Nutrition

Questions and Answers about Pregnancy

Questions and Answers about Complications

Crohn's Disease, Ulcerative Colitis and your
   Child

Coping with Crohn's Disease and Ulcerative
   Colitis (a booklet for children and
   teenagers)

Questions and Answers about Emotional
   Factors

A Teacher's Guide to Crohn's Disease and
   Ulcerative Colitis

Questions and Answers about Surgery

Books:

*Treating IBD: A Patient's Guide to the
   Medical and Surgical Management
   of Crohn's Disease,*
   Editors: Lawrence J. Brandt, M.D.,
   and Penny Steiner-Grossman, M.P.H.

*The New People . . . Not Patients:
   A Source Book for Living with IBD,*
   Editors: Penny Steiner-Grossman, M.P.H.,
   Peter A. Banks, M.D.,
   and Daniel H. Present, M.D.

*The Crohn's Disease and Ulcerative Colitis
   Fact Book,*
   Editors: Peter A. Banks, M.D.,
   Daniel H. Present, M.D.,
   and Penny Steiner, M.P.H.

The IBD Medical Record,
   Editor: Penny Steiner, M.P.H.

Magazine:
Foundation Focus

Fact Sheets ("IBD Files"):

Cigarette Smoking and Inflammatory Bowel
   Disease

Crohn's Disease Treatment Update:
   Metronidazole and 6-Mercaptopurine

Diagnostic Procedures and Laboratory Tests
   in IBD

Diagnostic X-Rays and IBD:
   Is There a Health Risk?

A Glossary of IBD Terms

How to Be a Hospital Visitor

IBD and the Emotions:
   Is There a Connection?

IBD and the Immune System

Inflammatory Bowel Disease and the Eyes

Inflammatory Bowel Disease:
   What Have We Learned?

New Drugs for IBD

New Surgeries for Ulcerative Colitis

Nutritional Support:
   When Food Is Not Enough

Nutrition and Inflammatory Bowel Disease

Obtaining Health Insurance

Questions and Answers about Cancer in IBD

Questions and Answers about IBD
   in Children

Questions and Answers about Recurrence
   in Crohn's Disease

Questions and Answers about Social Security
   Disability Insurance

Questions and Answers about Surgery
   in Crohn's Disease

The Search for an Infectious Agent in IBD

Treating the Arthritis of IBD

Treatment of Crohn's Disease with
   6-Mercaptopurine: A Long-Term,
   Randomized, Double-Blind Study

Treatment Update

What Is Lactose Intolerance?

Who Gets IBD?

Your Gastrointestinal Tract and How It Works

**For information on how to order any
of these publications, you may contact:**

The Crohn's & Colitis Foundation of
   America, Inc.
444 Park Avenue South
11th Floor
New York, NY 10016–7374

(212) 685-3440
(800) 343-3637 (Outside NY)
FAX: (212) 779-4098

Appendix B

Crohn's & Colitis
Foundation of America, Inc.

National Headquarters
444 Park Avenue South
11th Floor
New York, NY 10016–7374
(212) 685–3440
(800) 343–3637 (Outside NY)

Northeast Region I
94 Church Street
Suite 302
New Brunswick, NJ 08901
(908) 937–9100

Mid-Atlantic Region II
1314 Bedford Avenue
Suite 114
Baltimore, MD 21208
(410) 486–9511

Mid-West Region III
395 East Dundee Road
Suite 450
Wheeling, IL 60090
(708) 459–6342

South/Southwest Region IV
One Davis Boulevard
Suite 707
Tampa, FL 33606
(813) 251–2191

Western Region V
9740 Washington Boulevard
Culver City, CA 90232
(310) 559–8667

Southern California Region VI
4201 Wilshire Boulevard
Suite 624
Los Angeles, CA 90010
(213) 935–4673

Index

Israel, 3
IVP (*see* Intravenous pyelogram)

J

Jam, 119
Japan, 3
Jaundice, 89
Jejunoileitis, 21, 22
Jejunum, 21, 109
Jelly, 119
Jewish ancestry, 73
Jews, 64
Job (*see* Work)
Job applicants, 156, 157
Job loss, 149-150, 151, 158
Jogging, 133, 137
Joint pain, 20, 22, 26, 40, 106, 13
Jubelirer, Josh, 76
Junk foods, 108

K

Kidney function, 8, 43
Kidney stones, 9, 137
Kock pouch, 49
Konsyl,® 60
Kool-aid, 114
Kraft® Natural cheeses, 119
Kron, Audrey, 111, 125

L

Laboratory reports, 163
Laboratory tests, 7-18, 106, 161, 163, 166
Lack of interest, 82
Lactaid,® 116, 117
Lactase, 108, 109, 116
Lactose-free diet, 116-117
Lactose-free formulas, 115
Lactose intolerance, 108, 116
Lamb, 118, 119, 123
Late-onset, 93
Latin America, 140, 143
Law enforcement agencies, 161
Law school, 88
Laxatives, 9, 10, 15, 16, 56
Left-sided colitis (*see* Distal colitis)
Legumes, 121, 122, 123, 124
Leisure, 54
Lemonade, 118
Lentils, 121, 122, 123, 124
Life expectancy, 32, 67, 81, 96
Lifestyle, 131, 137
Lifetime maximum benefits, 151, 152
Light & Lively® cheeses, 119
Lignin, 118
Liquid diets, 114-115
Liquid foods, 135
Liquid formula supplements (*see also* Nutritional supplements), 109, 111, 120
Listlessness, 82
Lite Line® cheeses, 119
Liver as food, 121, 122, 123
Liver function, 8
Liver inflammation, 15
Lobster, 53, 123

Lomotil® (*see* Diphenoxylate)
Longevity (*see* Life expectancy)
Loop ileostomy, 58-59, 60
Loperamide, 45, 60, 91, 137, 142, 143
Loss of control, 29-33, 49, 65
Louisiana, 150, 152
Love, 82, 125, 127, 128, 129
Low-Fat diet, 118-120
Low-Residue/Low-Fiber diet, 117-118
Lumen, 4
Lymphocytes, 4

M

Macaroni, 116, 118
Macaroni and cheese, 121
Macrophages, 4
Magacal,® 116
Magazine (*see* Educational literature)
Magnesium, 118
Magnesium citrate, 16
Magnetic resonance imaging, 8, 13
Maine, 152, 158
Mainstreaming, 159
Maintenance therapy, 37, 40
Major-medical, 149, 150
Malabsorption, 21
Malaria, 140
Malnutrition (*see also* Nutritional status, Undernutrition), 9, 68, 111
"Managed care" programs, 149
Margarine, 110, 116, 117, 118, 119, 120, 121
Marijuana, 47
Marriage, 86, 127-128
Marshmallows, 56, 119
Massachusetts, 150
Mast cells, 4
Maximum coverage, 158
Mayonnaise, 118, 119
Meal size, 110
Meat, 113, 116, 118, 119, 120
Medicaid, 147, 152, 161
Medical history, 83, 93, 105, 150, 163, 165-166
Medical record, 105, 161-167
Medical Records: Getting Yours (Book), 166
Medical terminology, 165-166
Medicare, 147, 152, 161
Medications, 37-47, 77-78, 88-91, 100, 102, 105, 140
Mediterranean, 140
Medium-chain triglycerides, 110,120
Medrol® (*see* Methylprednisolone)
Melons, 52, 121
Menstruation, 107
Meperidine, 14, 47
6-Mercaptopurine, 42, 64, 90-91
Meringues, 119
Meritene,® 115
Mesalamine (*see* 5-Aminosalicylic acid)
Metallic taste, 44
Metamucil,® 17, 46, 60
Methotrexate, 44
Methylprednisolone, 41, 90
Metronidazole, 43, 61, 65, 66, 90
Mexico, 143
Michigan, 150
Microguard,® 61

Microscopic colitis, 94
Military hospitals, 164
Milk & milk products, 52, 78, 108, 109-110, 115, 116, 117, 118, 119, 120, 121, 122, 123
Milk shakes, 108, 120
Mineral deficiency, 7
Mineral sources, 122-124
Mineral water, 114, 141
Minerals, 107
Minnesota, 148, 152, 158
Mississippi, 150
Moisture barriers, 59, 61
Montana, 152
"Montezuma's revenge", 140
Moods, 125, 131
Morello, Valerie, 88
Morphine sulfate, 47
Mortality rate, 66-67
Motrin,® 95
Mouth, 20, 22
Mozzarella cheese, 117, 119, 124
6-MP (*see* 6-Mercaptopurine)
MRI (*see* Magnetic resonance imaging)
Mucins, 73
Muco-pus, 24, 26
Mucosa, 4, 5, 19, 23
Muenster cheese, 109, 124
Muscle weakness, 133
Mushrooms, 53
Mustard, 117
Mycolog,® 61
Mycostatin,® 61

N

Naprosyn,® 95
Narcotic bowel syndrome, 46
Narcotic dependence, 46-47
Narcotics, 45, 46, 140
Nasogastric feeding, 79, 86, 88, 110-111, 115
National health insurance, 153
National Parks, 139
National Research Council, 113
Native Americans, 64
Nausea, 9, 21, 38, 43, 44, 56, 77, 94, 128
NDA (*see* New Drug Application)
Nebraska, 150, 152
New Drug Application, 4, 5
New drugs, xi, 45, 104
New Drugs for IBD (Fact Sheet), 169
New Jersey, 148, 150, 158
New Mexico, 152
The New People...Not Patients: A Source Book for Living with IBD (Book), 169
New Surgeries for Ulcerative Colitis (Fact Sheet), 169
New York, 148
New Zealand, 140
Nitrogen, 114
Noodles, 110, 116, 118, 123
North Dakota, 150, 152
Nuclear medicine, 12
Numbness, 44, 46
Nursing (*see* Breast feeding)
Nursing care, 152
Nursing notes, 163, 166
Nutmeg, 117

Nutrament,® 115
Nutrient intake, 107, 108, 113
Nutrient loss, 107
Nutrition, 78-79, 87, 91, 107, 127, 134-135
Nutrition and Inflammatory Bowel Disease (Fact Sheet), 170
Nutritional requirements, 107, 109, 113
Nutritional standards, 3
Nutritional status (*see also* Malnutrition, Undernutrition), 8, 107, 110, 112, 115, 168
Nutritional supplements (*see also* Liquid formula supplements), 77, 79, 83, 86
Nutritional Support: When Food Is Not Enough (Fact Sheet), 170
Nutritional support program, 86, 91, 110, 113, 168
Nutritionist, 107, 112
Nuts, 53, 59, 110, 114, 119, 121, 123, 124

O

Obstruction (*see* Bowel obstruction)
Obtaining Health Insurance (Fact Sheet), 170
Occult blood, 8, 9, 21
Odor, 51-52
Office for Civil Rights, 160
Office visits, 99, 100-101, 102, 149
Oklahoma, 150
Okra, 53
Olbrisch, Mary Ellen, 65
Older adult, 93-96
Olsalazine, 40
Onions, 52
Onset of disease, 25, 26-27, 75, 93, 94, 95, 96, 106, 106
Operative pain (*see also* Pain), 30
Operative reports, 105, 163, 164
Opium, 47, 140
Orange juice, 118
Oranges, 121
Oregon, 152
Organ meats, 119
Osmolite,® 115, 116
Osteoporosis, 41, 66, 95
Ostomate, 54
    Definition, 51
Ostomy (*see also* Colostomy, Ileostomy), 31, 49-56, 83, 129, 136
Ostomy appliances, 29, 49, 57, 58, 92
    Definition, 51
Ostomy care, 59
Out-patient hospital services, 148, 150
Ova in stool, 8, 10
Ovaries, 87
Overprotectiveness, 80
Overseas travel, 140
Oxycodone, 47
Oysters, 121, 123

P

Pain (*see also* Abdominal pain, Chest pain, Joint pain, Operative pain), 31, 47, 56, 103, 125, 128
Pamphlets (*see* Educational literature)
Pancreatitis, 39, 40, 43, 66
Paprika, 117
Parasites in stool, 8, 9, 10

Parent-child communication, 76, 77
Parents (*see* Family members), 75-82, 83, 102, 130, 158
Parmesan cheese, 121
Parsley, 52, 121
Parsnips, 122
Pasta, 116, 119, 120, 121
Pastries, 116, 119
Pathology report, 163
Patient compliance, 27, 78, 103, 111
Patient education (*see also* Educational literature), 100
Patient-physician communication (*see* Physician-patient communication)
Patient rights, 162
Peaches, 121
Peanut butter, 54, 119, 120, 121
Peanuts, 121
Peas, 52, 53, 121, 122
Pectin, 118
Peers, 80
Pelvic nerve, 65
Pelvic scarring, 87
Penile erection, 89
Pennsylvania, 148
Pentazocaine, 47
Pepper, 117
Pepsin, 109
Peptamen,® 114
Pepti-2000,® 114
Pepto-Bismol,® 141
Percocet® (*see* Oxycodone)
Percodan® (*see* Oxycodone)
Perforation (*see* Bowel perforation)
Perianal disease (*see also* Perineal disease, Perirectal disease), 23, 44, 111, 137
Perianal irritation, 61
Perianal skin, 59, 60, 61
Pericarditis, 40
Peri-Care,® 59
Perineal disease (*see also* Perianal disease, Perirectal disease), 92
Perirectal disease (*see also* Perianal disease, Perineal disease), 23
Peristalsis, 50, 109
Peristomal skin, 52
Permission, 102
Personal account, 73, 76, 79, 84-85, 88, 111, 137
Personality change, 41
Phenothiazines, 45
Phosphorus, 114
Physical activity, 29, 133-135
Physical examination, 20, 105, 155, 163, 165
Physical impact, 99, 100
Physical needs, 29
Physical therapist, 138
Physician competence, 99, 103
Physician fees, 105, 152
Physician qualifications, 100
Physician roster, 100
Physician selection, 99, 100
Physician services, 150
Physician visits, 148
Physician-patient communication, 43, 83, 86, 99-106, 131, 139, 143
Physician-patient relationship, 15, 31, 32, 33, 99-106, 163

Pictorial representation, 77, 80, 100
Pie, 119
Pity, 131
Pizza, 108, 121, 122
Placenta, 89, 90
Plan of action, 143
Plaquenil® (*see* Hydroxychloroquine)
Platelet count, 8, 39, 43
Pneumonitis, 39, 40
Polycose,® 120
Popcorn, 59, 110, 114
Popsicles, 114
Pork, 110, 119, 123
Postoperative care, 103
Postoperative complications, 68
Postpartum period, 88
Pot pie, 121
Potassium, 114, 135, 138
Potato chips, 78
Potatoes, 110, 118, 120, 121, 123
Pouching systems, 58
"Pouchitis", 60-61
Poultry, 110, 116, 118, 119, 120
Precision Isotonic,® 114
Precision Low-Residue,® 114
Predisposition, 63, 72, 74
Prednisone, 7, 41, 64, 66, 77, 78, 79, 90, 110, 131, 143
Pre-existing conditions, 148, 151, 152, 158
Pregnancy, 39, 87-92, 129
Pregnancy outcome, 87
Pregnancy trimesters, 88, 90, 91, 92
Prematurity, 87, 90, 92
Prescription drugs, 152
Preventive health services, 148
Pretzels, 78, 116
Privacy, 101
Privacy Act of 1974, 106, 164
Proctitis (*see* Ulcerative proctitis)
Proctocolectomy, 57, 65, 89
Proctofoam-HC,® 41
Proctoscopy, 13
Proctosigmoiditis, 25, 26, 27, 39
Proctosigmoidoscopy, 13
Progress notes, 163
Prolapse of ileostomy, 92
Pro-mix,® 120
Propac,® 120
Prothrombin time, 8
Protein intake, 107, 108
Protein loss, 107, 114, 133, 135
Provolone cheese, 117
Prune juice, 117
Prunes, 123
Pseudopolyps, 24
Psychological counseling, 82, 103
Psychological factors, 127, 129
Psychotherapist, 125, 131
Psychotherapy, 130-131
Puberty, 81
Public accomodations, 156, 158
Public Citizen Health Research Group, 164
Public Health Service hospitals, 164
Puddings, 115, 118, 119, 121, 122
Puerto Rico, 139, 143
"Pull-through" operation, 49, 57-62, 66, 92, 95, 103